Immunological Investigation of Renal Disease

Immunological Investigation of Renal Disease

A. R. McGiven

M.D.(Otago), Ph.D.(Monash), F.R.C.P.A.
Professor and Chairman, Department of
Pathology, University of Otago, Christchurch
Clinical School of Medicine; Chairman of
Pathology Services, North Canterbury
Hospital Board, Christchurch, New Zealand.

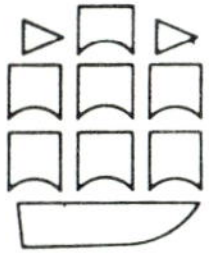

CHURCHILL LIVINGSTONE
EDINBURGH LONDON AND NEW YORK 1980

CHURCHILL LIVINGSTONE
Medical Division of the Longman Group Limited

Distributed in the United States of America by
Churchill Livingstone Inc., 19 West 44th Street,
New York, N.Y. 10036, and by associated companies,
branches and representatives throughout the world.

First published 1980

ISBN 0 443 01899 5

British Library Cataloguing in Publication Data
Immunological investigation of renal disease.
   1. Kidneys—Diseases   2. Immunology—
Technique
   I. McGiven, A R
   616.6'1'079028   RC903   79–40942

Printed in Great Britain by Butler & Tanner Ltd, Frome and London

Foreword

The explosive development of clinical immunology and the increasing breadth of its medical horizons during the last decade have outstripped the availability of practical texts to provide up-to-date information for hospital laboratory workers and clinicians. This has created a need for rapidly published specialized books detailing technical laboratory procedures and explaining their clinical relevance.

Practical Methods in Clinical Immunology should satisfy this need by providing a series of books dealing with individual body systems, or groups of diseases, or immunological events in disease. The range of topics so far decided is given in the accompanying 'In Preparation' list for the Series.

This first volume to appear, McGiven's *Immunological Investigation of Renal Disease*, is an excellent example of one such topic. Professor McGiven, with his colleagues, is well qualified for the task, having built up a new immunopathological laboratory during this last decade of clinical immunology growth, to provide an enviable high quality collaborative service for his clinical associates. In this book will be found practical details of immunological tests currently employed for investigating and treating renal disease, and a wealth of wisdom to help the nephrologist select appropriate tests and interpret their results.

Melbourne, 1980   R. C. N.

Preface

This book contains a wide-ranging selection of practical laboratory techniques which have been found to be useful in the immunological investigation and management of patients with renal disease.

Emphasis has been placed on providing detailed instructions so that the methods can be undertaken by laboratory workers with minimal reference to other sources. Wherever possible attention has been given to the interpretation of results and their clinical significance to assist physicians responsible for patient care.

In compiling this book I am indebted to my colleagues in the Pathology Services, Christchurch Hospital and in addition to fellow authors, Dr C. M. Andre, Mr J. S. Hunt and Miss Susan M. McQuilkan, and wish to thank the following who have assisted in a variety of ways with resource material: Mr W. A. Day (electron microscopy), Mr. K. McLoughlin (tissue typing), Mr. R. T. Fowler (total protein quantitation), Mr J. G. Lewis (S.D.S. polyacrylamide gel electrophoresis), Miss S. M. Lines (streptococcal antibodies) and Miss H. L. Martin, Mrs J. S. Eccersall, Dr K. E. Barber and Mr M. P. Kennedy (complement and immune complexes).

Special thanks are due to Mr K. A. Donaldson and the staff of the Department of Medical Illustration as well as to Mrs D. A. Laing who typed the manuscript.

I also wish to acknowledge the longstanding cooperation of Dr P. J. Little and Dr R. R. Bailey of the Department of Renal Medicine, Christchurch Hospital which has enabled us to gain experience in the investigation of renal disease.

Dr I. J. Simpson, School of Medicine, University of Auckland, provided helpful information on complement and immune complex procedures.

In conclusion, on behalf of all contributors, I wish to thank Professor R. C. Nairn, Series Editor, and the staff of Churchill Livingstone for their patience and assistance.

University of Otago, 1980   A. R. McG

Contributors

C. M. Andre
M.B., B.S.(Lond.), Head of Department of Clinical Biochemistry, Christchurch Hospital, Christchurch, New Zealand.

J. S. Hunt
M.Sc.(Cant.), M.N.Z.I.C. Hospital Scientific Officer, Department of Pathology, University of Otago, Christchurch Clinical School of Medicine, Christchurch, New Zealand.

A. R. McGiven
M.D.(Otago), Ph.D.(Monash), F.R.C.P.A. Professor of Pathology, University of Otago, Christchurch Clinical School of Medicine and the Chairman of Pathology Services, North Canterbury Hospital Board, Christchurch, New Zealand.

Susan M. McQuilkan
C.O.P.M.L.T., A.N.Z.I.M.L.T. Technologist in Charge of Protein Laboratory, Department of Clinical Biochemistry, Christchurch Hospital, Christchurch, New Zealand.

Contents

1
Introduction

A. R. McGiven

The immunological investigation of the patient suspected of having renal disease is a common clinical problem. In some cases the patient presents with symptoms such as haematuria, oedema, polyuria or anuria which clearly direct the physician's attention to renal investigations. In other cases the patient is not aware of a renal abnormality and may present with musculo-skeletal pain, signs of anaemia, or is found to have proteinuria or hypertension on routine clinical examination.

These symptoms direct attention to the patient's renal function and consideration of the usefulness of studies of the patient's plasma proteins including immunoglobulins, complement components and specific antibodies directed against microorganisms, particularly the streptococcus, or autoantibodies such as antinuclear antibodies.

Such investigations, undertaken in the full knowledge of the history and clinical state of the patient, may provide a strong indication of a diagnosis such as acute poststreptococcal glomerulonephritis, systemic lupus erythematosus, hypocomplementaemic mesangiocapillary glomerulonephritis, or multiple myeloma.

Examination of the urine remains an important investigation. The detection of protein and measurement of protein clearances provide diagnostic and prognostic information additional to that provided by microscopy and the usual biochemical tests. Selective proteinurias, which involve small molecular weight proteins, are more likely to improve with corticosteroid therapy than are non-selective proteinurias where the urine contains proteins with a wide range of molecular weights. Refinement of microbiological studies is also taking place and urine collection techniques have become more sophisticated as shown by the growing use of bladder puncture techniques in children.

Over the past two decades the increasing use of percutaneous needle biopsy of the kidney has yielded a wealth of morphological information and resulted in a plethora of classifications of glomerular disease. The addition of immuno-fluorescence techniques has provided a glimpse of the immunopathological processes occuring in the kidney and this has been amplified by the study of complement and other plasma factors. The recognition of conditions such as IgA nephropathy has resulted directly from the application of immunofluorescence techniques.

Many glomerular disorders, from their immunofluorescence patterns, appear to be associated with immune complex deposition and this has led to an increasing interest in the detection and analysis of immune complexes. The relationship of immune complexes in the blood to immunopathological events occurring in the kidney is often circumstantial and present tests do not detect specifically nephropathic complexes. In many cases the nature of the antigen concerned has not been determined and this remains a challenge to investigators.

Unfortunately, although many renal diseases resolve spontaneously or respond to therapy, a number of diseases arising from causes as diverse as the deposition of immune complexes, persisting infection, vesico-ureteric reflux or prolonged consumption of analgesics, do not respond or have reached a terminal stage by the time the patient presents to the physician. The prolongation of life in these cases by haemodialysis and renal transplantation has been a rewarding development in medical management in spite of economic considerations.

Renal transplantation can provide a worthwhile alternative to many patients where suitable donor kidneys are available. The science of tissue typing is making steady advances and the application of knowledge of the D locus and its related lymphocyte antigens and the typing of specific lymphocyte subpopulations hold promise of improved matching between donor and recipient. A start has been made into monitoring immunosuppression by a variety of immunological techniques with a view, if possible, to maintaining a constant level of suppression which is sufficient to prevent allograft rejection without unduly exposing the patient to the risk of overwhelming infection.

The growth of immunology as a laboratory discipline has been followed by its widespread application in almost all branches of medicine. Nowhere is this better illustrated than in the close relationship which immunology has developed with the field of nephrology. Not only are immunological processes intimately concerned with the basic cause of diseases such as glomerulonephritis but immunological methods are widely used in the investigation of diseases which do not have an immunological basis. Finally the renal transplant patient is a living example of the application of theoretical principles and practical immunological techniques.

The kidney is essentially a filter of plasma which not only may contain factors which cause damage to the kidney but also, by changes in its composition, reflects the functional effects of structural damage. It is appropriate that the next chapter considers plasma proteins and their measurement. Many practical hints are included in this section and these methods are referred to again in succeeding chapters, such is their importance in the routine diagnostic laboratory.

UNCITED BIBLIOGRAPHY

Albini B, Brentjens J R, Andres G A 1979 The Immunopathology of the Kidney. Arnold, London
Brenner B M, Hostetter T H, Humes H D 1978 Molecular basis of proteinuria of glomerular origin. New England Journal of Medicine 298: 826–833
Cameron J S, Williams D G 1977 Glomerulonephritis. Holborow E J & Reeves W G Immunology in Medicine. Academic Press, London, Grune & Stratton, New York, ch 17, p 581–629

McCluskey R T, Hall C L, Colvin R B 1978 Immune complex mediated diseases. Human Pathology 9: 71–84

Ting A, Williams K A, Morris P J 1978 Transplantation: Immunological monitoring. British Medical Bulletin 34: 263–270

Wilson C B 1977 Recent advances in the immunological aspects of renal disease. Federation Proceedings 36: 2171–2175

2

Plasma Proteins

C. M. Andre and Susan M. McQuilkan

Plasma contains a complex mixture of proteins of diverse origin and function. These may be broadly classified into two main functional groups, the carrier proteins and defence proteins listed in Table 2.1. In addition there are numerous

Table 2.1. Classification of major plasma proteins

Carrier proteins	Defence proteins
Albumin	Protease inhibitors *e.g.*
Lipoproteins	$\alpha 1$ antitrypsin and $\alpha 2$
Transferrin	macroglobulin
Haptoglobins	Complement
Haemopexin	Immunoglobulins
Ceruloplasmin	Coagulation factors
Carriers of hormones and vitamins	Fibrinolysins

circulating tissue proteins, enzymes, polypeptide and protein hormones in varying but smaller amounts.

The plasma proteins are in dynamic equilibrium with the proteins of the extravascular fluids and tissues. In healthy adults the concentration of the various plasma proteins in an individual, remains relatively constant over long periods of time due to the balance between synthesis, distribution and catabolism. In disease states deviations from the normal plasma concentrations become apparent. The changes may be restricted to one protein, a group of proteins or be nonspecific affecting all plasma proteins. An increase in the plasma concentration of a single protein or group of proteins is usually the result of increased synthesis rather than reduced catabolism but a general increase of all plasma proteins indicates a reduction in plasma volume. A decrease in plasma protein concentrations may be the result of congenital or acquired defects of synthesis, increased catabolism or abnormal losses. Inherited defects of synthesis usually affect a single protein but abnormal losses commonly involve many different plasma proteins.

The analysis of plasma proteins by electrophoresis and specific protein quantitation provides valuable diagnostic hints on the presence, progression and complication of disease. For example excessive glomerular protein losses result in a typical plasma protein pattern referred to later. The acute phase proteins $\alpha 1$-antitrypsin, orosomucoid, haptoglobin and fibrinogen react as a group to an inflammatory process producing characteristic patterns. Immunoglobulin abnormalities may point *e.g.* to an autoimmune process or lymphoproliferative disorder. For further information on this topic the reader is referred to the publication by Laurell et al (1975).

In immunologic renal diseases the defence proteins, in particular immunoglobulins, complement and fibrinogen are of prime interest. A brief review of the immunoglobulins follows.

IMMUNOGLOBULINS

Immunoglobulin molecules consist of two pairs of identical polypeptide chains held together by disulphide bonds and non-covalent hydrophobic interactions. The larger or heavy (H) chains may be one of five types—γ, α, μ, δ or ε and confer class and sub-class specificity on the immunoglobulin molecule. The smaller light (L) chains which are shared by all immunoglobulin classes, may be of κ or λ types but are of the same type within an individual immunoglobulin molecule. The position of inter-H-L chain disulphide bonds and inter-H chain disulphide bonds is variable depending upon the class and sub-class of immunoglobulins. Intra-chain disulphide bonds are however relatively constant.

Comparison of the amino acid sequence analysis of monoclonal immunoglobulins has revealed that H and L chains contain variable and constant regions (Fig. 2.1). The carboxy-terminal half of L chains show two main sequence patterns with little variability within each pattern, corresponding to the κ and λ type of L chains. Allotypic differences have been demonstrated within the constant region of the κ chain. Much greater variability is found in the amino-terminal halves of L chains. In H chains within a given sub-class, apart from the variable amino-terminal segment (V), the remainder of the sequences are identical except for allotypic substitutions. These genetic markers are inherited by individuals as co-dominant factors. The constant region of H chains (C) can be subdivided into equal homologous regions or domains numbered C_H1 to

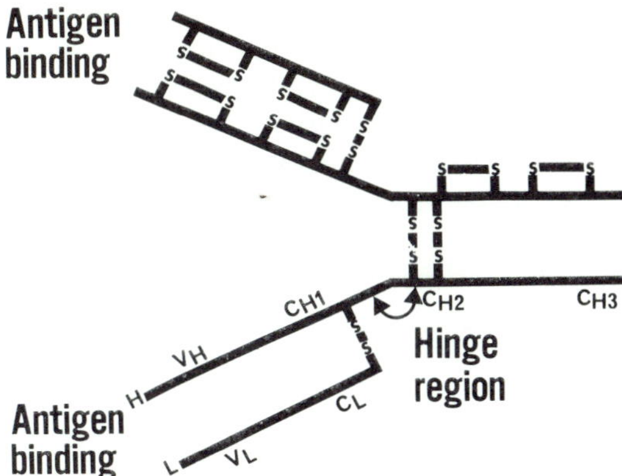

Figure 2.1. Diagram of immunoglobulin molecule showing heavy (H) and light (L) chains with variable (V) and constant (C) regions. The domains on the constant portion of the heavy chain are numbered C_H1, C_H2, C_H3. (IgM and IgE have an additional constant domain). Inter- and intra- chain disulphide bonds —S—S— are shown; omitted on the lower half of the molecule for clarity.

C_H4. The C_H regions provide the molecular basis for the different functional and metabolic characteristics of the various immunoglobulin classes. It is also noteworthy that L chains of κ type predominate in immunoglobulins, but the κ to λ ratio varies according to immunoglobulin class, age of subject, ethnic group and in diseases.

Immunoglobulin of γ class, IgG, is the major immunoglobulin component in plasma and consists of four subtypes IgG_1, IgG_2, IgG_3, IgG_4, which occur in the following proportion, 75 : 15 : 7 : 3. The biological properties of the sub-types vary e.g. only IgG_1 and IgG_3 immune complexes activate complement by the classical pathway. IgG is equally distributed between the blood and extra-vascular compartment. In the context of immunological renal disease it is the immunoglobulin most frequently identified in glomerular deposits.

Immunoglobulin of μ class, IgM, occurs in plasma primarily as a pentamer with an additional small polypeptide chain, the J chain. Monomeric IgM is also found in small amounts in normal plasma and in higher concentration in sera from patients with a variety of diseases. IgM is a predominantly intravascular immunoglobulin accounting for 80% of the total amount. It has strong agglutinating properties and bound to an antigen is a very efficient activator of the classical complement pathway. Circulating antibodies to immunoglobulins *i.e.* rheumatoid factor are usually but not exclusively of the IgM class. In immune complex nephropathies IgM may accompany IgG and IgA but in some types of glomerular lesions it is the only immunoglobulin component found.

Immunoglobulin of α class, IgA, occurs in plasma mainly in the monomeric form, however dimers, trimers and higher polymers are found. These polymeric forms also contain one J chain per molecule. IgA is the principal immuno-globulin in exocrine secretions such as intestinal and respiratory secretions, tears, saliva and milk. The IgA of secretion occurs chiefly as a dimer containing a J chain and an additional polypeptide chain, the secretory component probably produced by the epithelial cells lining the mucosal surface. The IgA molecule acquires the secretory component during transit across the epithelial surface. The function of the secretory component is unknown but it may stabilize and protect secretory IgA from digestion or other adverse conditions in secretions. IgM found in secretions also contains a complexed secretory component. Secre-tory IgA belongs mostly to the IgA_2 class whereas plasma IgA belongs mostly to the IgA_1 class. Most but not all IgA_2 molecules lack the inter-H and -L chain disulphide bond characteristic of all other immunoglobulins. In some types of glomerular immune deposits, *e.g.* IgA nephropathy and Henoch Schönlein pur-pura, IgA is the predominant immunoglobulin component.

Immunoglobulin of δ class, IgD, forms less than 1% of total plasma immunoglobulins and no major function or involvement in renal disease has yet been demonstrated.

Immunoglobulin of ε class, IgE, is concerned in reaginic cell bound activity associated with allergic phenomena, where antigen reacts with antibody bound to the surface of mast cells and leads to the release of pharmacologically active agents. It is present in very low concentrations in plasma. A defined role for IgE in renal lesions awaits demonstration.

Immunoglobulins have varied functions but in a nutshell as described by

Table 2.2. Physicochemical properties of immunoglobulins

Class	IgG	IgA	IgM	IgD	IgE
Molecular formula	$\gamma 2\ \kappa 2$	$(\alpha 2\ \kappa 2)n$	$(\mu 2\ \kappa 2)_5$	$\delta 2\ \kappa 2$	$\varepsilon 2\ \kappa 2$
	or	or	or	or	or
	$\gamma 2\ \lambda 2$	$(\alpha 2\ \lambda 2)n$	$(\mu 2\ \lambda 2)_5$	$\delta 2\ \lambda 2$	$\varepsilon 2\ \lambda 2$
Mean molecular weight	150 000	(160 000)n	900 000	178 000	187 000
Antigen binding sites	2	2	5–10	2	2
Rate of synthesis (mg/kg/d)	30	24	7	0.4	0.02
Plasma half life (d)	23	6	5	3	2
Plasma concentration (g/l)	7–13	0.8–3.5	0.6–2.0	< 0.03	< 0.00003

Hobbs (1971), IgG protects the body fluids, IgA protects the body surfaces, IgM protects the bloodstream, and IgE mediates reaginic hypersensitivity. The physicochemical properties of immunoglobulins are summarized in Table 2.2.

Immunoglobulins in renal disease

Changes in plasma immunoglobulin concentrations are influenced by a number of factors, and in renal disease the picture may be complicated by proteinuria, resulting in low plasma levels of IgG, and by the effects of uraemia. Renal failure can effect a toxic inhibition of synthesis affecting primarily IgM, then IgA and lastly IgG.

It is noteworthy that an elevation of IgG increases its catabolism. A subnormal level of IgG may be the result of increased catabolism or decreased synthesis whereas in most instances decreased IgA and IgM are due to impaired synthesis. It should also be borne in mind that the antibody response to an antigenic challenge varies both qualitatively and quantitatively. Some antigens *e.g.* lipopolysaccharides appear to stimulate bursal lymphocytes (B cells) without requiring the intervention of thymic lymphocytes (T cells). Characteristically thymus-independent antigens provoke an IgM response with little or no secondary IgG response. Whereas an antigen driven, T cell-dependent response, results in the appearance in the circulation of antibodies in the following class order, IgM, IgG and IgA. It should also be appreciated that potent antibodies against cells may be formed which might be undetectable by the ordinary assay methods for immunoglobulins.

Some diseases are associated with particular patterns of plasma immunoglobulin concentrations. Most of these patterns, however, lack specificity and the interested reader is referred to Hobbs (1971) for further information. A special case is the detection of monoclonal immunoglobulins and/or components when important diagnostic information may be obtained.

The interpretation of reported levels of immunoglobulins or other plasma proteins requires consideration of a number of factors listed below.

(*i*) Genetic.
(*ii*) Physiological, *e.g.* age, sex, nutrition, posture.
(*iii*) Metabolic, *e.g.* rates of synthesis and clearance, distribution in the body compartments.

(*iv*) Environmental, *e.g.* seasonal changes, geographic location.
 (*v*) Duration of disease and effect of intercurrent disease or infection.
(*vi*) Complication of disease, *e.g.* protein loss, changes in blood volume.
(*vii*) Treatment, *e.g.* drugs such as corticosteroids, diazoxide and phenytoin. The latter may produce a selective IgA deficiency.
(*viii*) Technical. Pitfalls are abundant and are discussed in the section on methods.

In the context of immunologically determined renal disease it is often more informative to detect specific antibodies (*e.g.* antistreptolysin 0 antibodies, antiDNA antibodies, antiglomerular basement membrane antibodies), circulating immune complexes and the deposition of immunoglobulins and complement in renal tissues, than to measure plasma immunoglobulins according to class.

The quantitation of changes in complement levels consequent upon activation of the immune response and fibrinogen degradation also provides useful diagnostic information. These investigations will be considered in subsequent chapters. The value of measuring the relative renal clearances of immunoglobulins to other proteins is discussed in Chapters 6 and 8.

PROTEIN ANALYSES

Protein analyses of both serum and urine provide helpful information about patients with renal disease. Choice of technique depends on the nature of the renal disorder being investigated; the application of each technique is discussed under its specific heading.

TOTAL PROTEIN QUANTITATION

The quantitation of total plasma proteins alone is usually unhelpful, except to demonstrate excessive fluctuations in levels, because of the independent changes in the concentration of specific proteins. Plasma protein levels must be considered, when assessing the clinical significance of proteinuria. It is also essential to know the plasma protein level when using quantitative zone electrophoresis. Electrophoresis and specific protein quantitation will provide more helpful information.

Estimation of total protein

Serum is mixed with biuret reagent and a coloured complex is formed between cupric ions and peptide bonds in a moderately alkaline medium. The colour which develops is compared with a protein standard. A correction for the sample blank is included.

Specimen
A fasting blood sample is drawn with minimal haemostasis and transferred into a plain collecting tube and allowed to stand until it has clotted spontaneously. After centrifugation, the serum is drawn off. Alternatively, heparinized

plasma may be used. Specimens are stored at 4°C. For prolonged storage, specimens should be frozen.

Reagents

NaOH 6M. Dissolve 240 g NaOH in distilled water and dilute to 1 litre. Store at ambient temperature in a tightly closed polyethylene bottle.

Biuret reagent. Dissolve 3 g ($\pm$ 0.01 g) $CuSO_4.5H_2O$ in 500 ml of distilled water. Add 9 g ($\pm$ 0.01 g) K, Na-tartrate and 5 g of KI. When completely dissolved, add 100 ml of 6M NaOH and dilute to 1 litre with distilled water. Store at ambient temperature in a tightly closed polyethylene bottle. It is important to make the reagent in the order as described to avoid precipitation.

Blank biuret reagent. Dissolve 9 g K, Na-tartrate and 5 g KI in distilled water. Add 100 ml 6M NaOH and dilute to 1 litre with distilled water. Store at ambient temperature in a tightly closed polyethylene bottle.

NaCl/NaN₃ solution. Dissolve 9 g NaCl and 0.50 g NaN_3 in 1 litre of distilled water.

Protein standard 80 g/l. A 'standard reference material' total protein standard (bovine serum albumin) issued by the U.S. National Bureau of Standards is used as the primary standard to determine the concentration of the secondary standard which is a human or bovine serum albumin. Suitable material is available from: Dade Company (8% Human Albumin Crystallized); Sigma Company (Bovine Albumin 100 g/l); Commonwealth Serum Laboratories (Human Albumin 250 g/l).

The biuret procedure as detailed in this communication is used in standardizing other protein solutions against the primary standard. The appropriately standardized secondary standard is diluted to 80 g/l with the $NaCl/NaN_3$ solution.

Quality control. A number of suitable commercial lyophilized sera are available.

Method

    (*i*) Pipette into test tubes, the serum sample, quality control serum and protein standard as follows:

	Test	Blank
Serum sample	0.1 ml	0.1 ml
Quality control serum	0.1 ml	0.1 ml
Protein standard 80 g/l	0.1 ml	0.1 ml

  (*ii*) To each test add 5.0 ml of biuret reagent. Mix.

  (*iii*) To each blank add 5.0 ml of blank biuret reagent. Mix.

  (*iv*) Prepare a reagent blank by mixing 0.1 ml of distilled water with 5.0 ml of biuret reagent.

  (*v*) Stand tubes at ambient temperature for 30 min.

  (*vi*) Measure the absorbance (A) of the reagent blank and tests at 540 nm in 10 mm cuvettes with distilled water as reference. Measure the absorbance of the blanks at the same wavelength with the blank biuret reagent as reference.

Calculation.

$$\frac{\text{(A) sample test}-\text{(A) reagent blank}+\text{sample blank}}{\text{(A) standard test}-\text{(A) reagent blank}+\text{standard blank}}\times 80 = \text{g/l}$$

Reference range. A suggested adult reference range is 65–80 g/l. Laboratories should determine their own reference range.

Note.

(*i*) Laboratories should check that Beer's Law is obeyed by setting up a series of standards within the range 0 to 140 g/l.

(*ii*) The biuret reagent should be discarded if any signs of precipitate are seen. Monitoring the absorbance at 540 nm may point to deterioration of the biuret reagent.

(*iii*) It is desirable that the protein content of the quality control sample be significantly different from the protein standard to highlight possible standardization errors.

(*iv*) Lipaemic, haemolysed, icteric sera and drugs in specimens may give erroneous results.

INDIVIDUAL PROTEIN ANALYSES

Agarose gel electrophoresis

Separation of proteins by electrophoresis is a valuable analytical tool for identifying serum protein patterns associated with disease. Agarose gel electrophoresis is a simple, effective technique, which allows the simultaneous separation of many samples (15 with our equipment). The method is suitable for clinical routine analyses of proteins in serum and other body fluids; a high degree of resolution is obtained resulting in patterns which are easy to interpret.

Agarose is a non-convective support medium, superior to cellulose acetate, giving better resolution and allowing separation of up to 16 protein fractions. Genetic variants and abnormal proteins, are more readily detected on agarose than on cellulose acetate.

Equipment

See Equipment for Protein Analyses

Direct current power supply—Electrophoretic chamber—Wettex strips 200 × 20 × 3 mm.—Levelling table.

Magnetic stirrer hot plate—Glass plate 205 × 110 × 1.5 mm—Slit former, rectangular teeth 0.5 mm.

Beakers for dispensing agarose: 50 ml; 200 ml. 3 μl automatic pipette.

Weight approximately 2 kg for pressing.—31 ET chromatography paper.—Oven at 90°C.

Reagents

(*i*) *Electrophoresis buffer.* Tris-veronal-sodium veronal buffer, 0.1 M pH 8.8:

Veronal-sodium	9.5 g	
Veronal	3.0 g	Make up to 1 litre with
Tris	4.6 g	distilled water.
Calcium lactate	0.4 g	

The addition of calcium ions improves the resolution of the protein fractions. By changing the polarity after each successive electrophoresis, the buffer can tolerate approximately 10 electrophoretic runs.

(*ii*) *Fixing solution.* Saturated solution of picric acid in distilled water mixed 3:1 with glacial acetic acid. The picric acid mixture should not be reused for more than 15 gel plates, as the ability of the mixture to fix the proteins is reduced with time and use.

(*iii*) *Staining solution.* Amido Black B 5 g/l or Coomassie Brilliant Blue R-250, 5 g/l in an ethanol (0.96 by vol.)—glacial acetic acid—water mixture, in the proportion 9:2:9. The stain is dissolved in the ethanol—acetic acid—water mixture and allowed to mix for 24 h prior to filtering through Whatman No 1. Coomassie Brilliant Blue R-250 is the protein stain of choice being at least three times more sensitive than Amido Black B; it is stable and can be restored at room temperature.

(*iv*) *Destaining solution.* Ethanol (0.96 by vol.)—glacial acetic acid—water mixture in the proportion 9:2:9. The solution is stable and may be made in large volumes.

(*v*) *Diluent for serum proteins.* Tris-veronal-sodium veronal buffer 0.2 M containing 300 ml glycerol/l buffer, and 1 g/l Bromphenol Blue. Bromphenol Blue binds to albumin, thus allowing the albumin front to be followed during electrophoresis. The glycerol increases the density of the sample thereby reducing the speed at which it diffuses out of the well and allowing the sample to move evenly into the agarose.

(*vi*) *Agarose.* The choice of agarose is of major importance when considering electrophoretic techniques. Miles Seravac or BDH are suitable sources; their agarose is optically clear with moderate gelling properties. The content of negatively charged groups gives moderate to high electroendosmosis. A highly purified agarose may not achieve adequate electroendosmosis needed to facilitate the migration of the gamma globulins.

Method
Preparation of agarose gel plate. (Approximately 1.0 mm in thickness). Agarose 50 ml of 10 g/l in tris-veronal buffer 0.1 M is boiled in an Erlenmeyer flask on a magnetic stirrer hot plate. A glass filter funnel approximately 40 mm in diameter is placed in the neck of the flask to reduce water loss during boiling. Care should be taken to avoid overheating and charring of agarose. The agarose must be completely dissolved in the boiling buffer before the plate is poured. To pour plate—

(*i*) Rinse 50 ml beaker in tap water 60°C and place in 200 ml beaker containing tap water 60°C.

(*ii*) Pipette precisely 25 ml of molten agarose into the 50 ml beaker.

(*iii*) Preheat a clean, grease free glass plate in 90°C oven and place on levelling table.

(*iv*) Quickly but gently pour molten agarose onto middle of glass plate. Obtain an even thickness of gel by spreading agarose from centre to edge of plate with a glass rod.

(*v*) Immediately the plate is poured position slit former approximately 5 mm from longer edge of plate and allow to set for 20 min.

Preparation and application of serum samples. Samples to be electrophoresed should differ as little as possible in ionic strength and pH from the gel buffer. Serum samples and a control are thus diluted 1:1 in the glycerol-tris-veronal diluent. 3 μl of diluted samples and a control are applied to the slits by micro-automatic pipette, immediately after the removal of the slit former. The sample should be level with the gel surface without overflowing. Any liquid in the wells must be removed before application of the samples by gently touching the slit surface with torn filter paper. It is essential that the slits are not damaged in any way to avoid poor quality electrophoresis.

Separation of proteins by electrophoresis. The prepared plate is carefully placed on the water cooled support bridge of the electrophoretic chamber. To ensure efficient cooling of the gel, a thin water film, without air bubbles, is retained between the glass plate and the cooling surface. Some workers have found that the use of 0.5 g/l non-ionic detergent on the support bridge reduces trapping of air bubbles. Contact is made between the gel plate and buffer by means of Wettex strips via the agarose bridges, the strips having been moistened with electrophoresis buffer. Electrophoresis is performed with a high potential gradient of 20 V/cm and a cooling water temperature of 10–15°C, corresponding to 250–260 V across the plate and a current of 100–120 mA. It is important that the potential gradient is balanced against the cooling efficiency of the system: too intense cooling or insufficient cooling will distort the electrophoretic pattern. Electrophoresis is stopped when the albumin front is approximately 10 mm from the edge of the anodal Wettex strip, taking an average time of 55 min. Ensure that the power supply is turned off before removing the plate from the electrophoretic chamber.

Fixation and staining of separated proteins. The separated proteins are fixed in saturated picric acid solution for 10 min. The gel is then covered with a layer of 31 ET chromatography paper avoiding air bubbles; soft paper is essential. The gel layer is reduced to a thin film by placing several layers of paper towels and a 3 mm thick glass plate on top and pressing with a 2 kg weight for 15 min. The plate is then completely dried at 90°C with chromatography paper on the gel. The chromatography paper is removed and the plate washed free of excess picric acid with cold tap water. The protein fractions are stained in Coomassie Brilliant Blue for at least 10 min, washed with cold tap water and then destained for approximately 30 s to remove excess dye. Avoid over destaining. The plate is washed again in cold tap water and oven-dried. A photograph of the plate provides a record.

Technical comments

(*i*) Agarose bridge and electrophoresis buffer should be changed after 10 electrophoretic runs and the entire electrophoretic chamber should be washed with tap water and reassembled.

(*ii*) Between electrophoretic runs ensure that the Wettex strips are kept in their respective buffer vessels in the electrophoretic chamber. When the electrophoretic chamber is being cleaned the Wettex strips are rinsed thoroughly and boiled in tap water before being returned to the buffer vessels.

(*iii*) A fasting serum sample is preferred for some electrophoretic analyses, as the fibrinogen band visualized in plasma samples may obscure an underlying monoclonal immunoglobulin. However, Laurell is in favour of blood being collected directly into Na_2 EDTA because fewer proteases are activated, resulting in greater sample stability for the labile C3 and C4 components. The increase in α and β lipoprotein mobility with sample aging is also reduced. Furthermore fibrinogen abnormalities may be detected.

(*iv*) The proteins in other body fluids such as urine and cerebrospinal fluid are also satisfactorily separated on agarose gel after suitable concentration of the sample.

(*v*) Sample collection requires care. For serum avoid prolonged venous stasis and haemolysis. For urine and other body fluids, samples should be as fresh as possible and preferably free of preservatives.

(*vi*) Storage of samples is normally satisfactory in stoppered polyethylene, polycarbonate or glass tubes at 4°C for at least one week. For longer periods of time, samples should be stored frozen. Repeated thawing and freezing of samples should be avoided at all times as this denatures proteins. Some workers prefer to preserve samples with sodium azide at a concentration of 1 g/l. Azides form unstable, explosive complexes with copper and other metals and care should be taken to dispose of azide-containing fluids in appropriate drainage outlets.

(*vii*) The separated protein fractions are examined visually without quantitation. The patient's protein patterns are compared with a serum pool of at least seven healthy hepatitis B negative male donors, and a fresh dilution of the pool is used each day.

Interpretation of serum protein patterns on agarose gel
Qualitative serum protein electrophoresis provides most information when the protein patterns are interpreted in conjunction with selected specific protein quantitation and clinical findings. Differences in the electrophoretic pattern of healthy individuals may be due to genetic variants, age-dependent changes in concentration, physiological states *e.g.* pregnancy, or medication *e.g.* oral contraceptives.

Electrophoretic patterns are analysed by comparing each horizontal row of bands and looking for—

(*i*) changes in concentration of individual protein fractions or protein groups;
(*ii*) heterogeneity of a protein fraction;
(*iii*) variation in protein mobility;
(*iv*) presence of abnormal discrete bands.

Commonly encountered abnormal electrophoretic patterns (Cf. normal Fig. 2.2) are shown in Figs. 2.3 to 2.6.

Acute phase reaction. (Fig. 2.3). The protein pattern observed is a manifestation of an inflammatory process. The intensity and type of response depends on its nature and duration. Typically there is a decrease in albumin with an increase

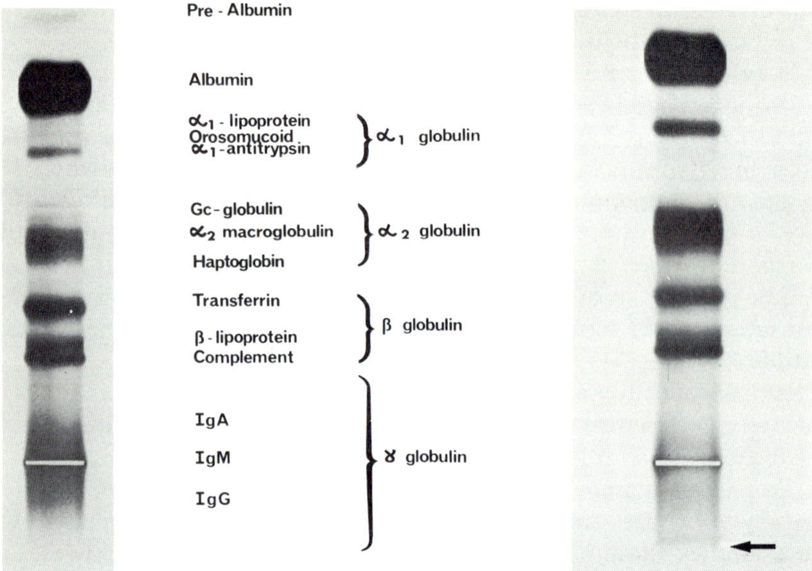

Figure 2.2. Normal serum protein electrophoresis in agarose gel. Complement refers to C3.
Figure 2.3. Serum electrophoretic pattern showing typical acute phase reaction with decrease in albumin, increase in αl and α2 globulins and C-reactive protein (arrow).

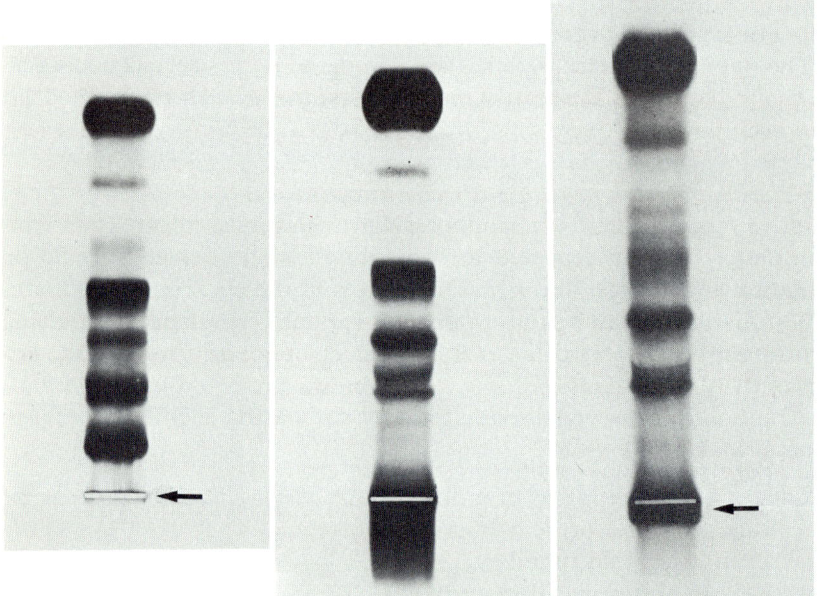

Figure 2.4. Typical plasma protein electrophoretic pattern in nephrotic syndrome. Albumin and γ globulins reduced, α2 globulin, β-lipoprotein and fibrinogen elevated. Fibrinogen band located between β-lipoprotein and origin (arrow).
Figure 2.5. Serum protein electrophoretic pattern showing polyclonal increase in γ globulins and increased α2 globulin fraction.
Figure 2.6. Abnormal discrete band indicated by arrow subsequently identified by immunoelectrophoresis as a monoclonal immunoglobulin.

in αl globulin (orosomucoid and αl antitrypsin), α2 globulin (haptoglobin) and C-reactive protein. Later, a gradual increase in complement and immunoglobulins may be seen.

Nephrotic syndrome. (Fig. 2.4). This is characterized by marked proteinuria, hypoproteinaemia, oedema and commonly hyperlipidaemia. There is a common feature, namely excessive loss of low molecular weight proteins through the glomeruli with retention of higher molecular weight proteins. This results in a typical nephrotic pattern characterized by marked decrease in albumin, increase in α2 macroglobulin, β-lipoprotein and fibrinogen and often decrease in immunoglobulins.

Hypergammaglobulinaemia
Polyclonal increase in gammaglobulins (Fig. 2.5) is due to the stimulation of numerous plasma cell clones by either exogenous or endogenous antigens. This broad, diffuse, heterogeneous increase in the gammaglobulin fraction is associated with a number of clinical disorders due to chronic infection, autoimmune disease, chronic liver disease and others such as neoplasms and sarcoidosis. Associated tissue damage or renal disorder with nephrotic syndrome will be manifested by the appropriate plasma protein changes.

Monoclonal disorder (Fig. 2.6) is characterized by a discrete immunoglobulin (and/or component) band as in multiple myeloma, in which case immunosuppression, manifested by a reduction in the other immunoglobulins is often observed. Monoclonal immunoglobulins may in certain instances, appear nondiscrete, presenting problems in their detection. When this occurs, it is usually monoclonal IgA, IgM or heavy chain components. The mobility of some monoclonal immunoglobulins and monoclonal light chains, *i.e.* Bence-Jones protein, may be such that they are superimposed on another protein fraction, causing the fraction, *e.g.* complement or transferrin, to appear intensely stained. Kappa light chains may also bind to αl antitrypsin and some other proteins.

There are several protein fractions which will mimic monoclonal immunoglobulins and Bence-Jones protein. When pseudomonoclonal proteins are suspected, the Ouchterlony double diffusion method provides a rapid means of identification and may prevent the need for further investigations such as immunoelectrophoresis or crossed immunoelectrophoresis. Some of the proteins which may mimic monoclonal immunoglobulins are listed in Table 2.3.

Table 2.3. Proteins mistaken for monoclonal immunoglobulins

Electrophoretic mobility	Protein component
Albumin	Bisalbumin
Alpha 1	Alpha fetoprotein
	Alpha 1 antitrypsin variants
Beta	Transferrin variants
	Complement degradation products
	Beta lipoprotein
Beta Gamma	Fibrinogen
	Bacterial contamination
Gamma	C-reactive protein
	Muramidase (lysozyme)

Ouchterlony double diffusion

Antigen and antibody simultaneously diffuse towards each other through agarose gel. The antigen-antibody complex formed at equivalence is visualized as a white precipitin line between the wells. The Ouchterlony double-immunodiffusion technique is at best semiquantitative and lends itself primarily to qualitative tests for the presence and characterization of specific proteins such as C-reactive protein and fibrinogen. It also provides a simple and direct method for determining whether antigenic determinants are identical, partially identical or non-identical. For further details see Ouchterlony & Nilsson (1978).

Equipment

Magnetic stirrer hot plate—Levelling table—Glass plate, approximately 60 × 40 × 2 mm—4.0 mm telescopic gel puncher—10 µl automatic pipette—Humidifier—Light box.

Reagents

(*i*) *Tris-veronal-sodium veronal buffer* (0.1 M, pH 8.8). *See* Agarose Gel Electrophoresis buffer.

(*ii*) *Agarose.* Miles Seravac—10 g/l.

(*iii*) *Antisera.* Rabbit anti-human sera to the specific proteins to be investigated.

Method

Preparation of agarose gel plate (1.0–2.0 mm in thickness). Molten agarose is prepared in a manner similar to that for agarose gel electrophoresis. To pour plate.—

(*i*) Place warmed glass plate on levelling table.

(*ii*) Spread 6 ml of molten agarose evenly across the plate.

(*iii*) The agarose should be left to gel for at least 10 min before punching the wells.

Punching of wells. Wells, 4.0 mm in diameter, are punched by means of a telescopic gel puncher at appropriate positions on the gel plate. The positioning of the wells is dependent on the investigation required. A distance of 4–5 mm is generally adequate separation between wells. Before application of antigen and antibody, to prevent diffusion under the gel, the bottom of each well is sealed with a drop of molten agarose.

Application of antigen and antibody. Equal volumes, *e.g.* 10 µl of antigen and antibody are applied to the respective wells. It is advisable to use positive and negative control samples.

Diffusion. The gel plate is placed in a humidifier at room temperature, for a time dependent on the specific antigen-antibody system under investigation, *e.g.* 1–72 h.

Reading of results. The white precipitin lines formed at equivalence of antigen to antibody are best visualized against a dark background with oblique lighting. The results may be recorded by pressing the gel and staining as for immuno-electrophoresis, after which a photograph is taken.

Technical comments
Samples. Proteins present in serum, plasma, cryoprecipitates and urine may be identified by the Ouchterlony double-diffusion technique.

Glass plates must be scratch free, to permit clear reading of precipitin lines.

Temperature. Diffusion is satisfactory at temperatures ranging from 18–37°C. The diffusion rate of antigens and antibodies is accelerated by increase in temperature. Temperature changes should be avoided because they may distort the immunoprecipitates.

Artefacts in immunoprecipitation may also be caused by defects in wells or denaturation of antibody or antigen during migration.

Sensitivity of the Ouchterlony technique is dependent on distance between the wells, concentration of reactants and concentration and thickness of gel. Concentration of antigens greater than 2 mg/l have been detected by this technique.

Sources of error. (*i*) Excessive amounts of antigen or antibody may inhibit visible immunoprecipitation. To ensure that equivalence of antigen to antibody is reached, serial dilutions of the antigen or antiserum are made and applied to the appropriate wells. (*ii*) Aged or lipaemic samples may produce circular precipitates around the antigen wells. (*iii*) Sometimes more than one immunoprecipitin line may form because of heterogeneity of antibodies and antigenic determinants present or interaction between antisera.

Electroimmunoassay (Laurell rockets)

Particular proteins such as immunoglobulins, albumin, transferrin and complement components, which are frequently affected by renal disease, may be quantitated by electroimmunoassay. Antigen is electrophoresed into an agarose gel containing monospecific antisera. The eventual height of the rocket-shaped precipitate formed at equivalence of antigen to antibody, is proportional to the concentration of the antigen.

Equipment
See Equipment for Protein Analyses.

Direct current power supply—Electrophoretic chamber—Wettex strips 200 × 20 × 3 mm—Magnetic stirrer hot plate—Two glass plates, 205 × 110 × 1.5 mm—One U-frame, 205 × 110 × 1.0 mm—Four bulldog clips—50 ml fine-lipped measuring cylinder—2.5 mm telescopic gel puncher—Gel punching template—3 μl automatic pipette—Dialysis tubing (optional)—Thermometer 0–110°C—Weight approximately 2 kg for pressing—31 ET chromatography paper—Oven at 90°C—Ruler graduated in mm.

Reagents
Electrophoresis buffer. Veronal-glycine-tris buffer (pH 8.8, ionic strength 0.08), prepared by mixing equal volumes of Buffer 1 and Buffer 2 before use. Buffer 1: veronal-Na—13 g; veronal—2.07 g; dissolved in 1 litre distilled water. Buffer 2: glycine—56.2 g; Tris—42.2 g; dissolved in 1 litre distilled water.

Agarose. (*i*) Litex HSA 15 g/l; (*ii*) Miles-Seravac 10 g/l. Agarose with a low electroendosmotic flow is preferable as the antibodies in the gel should remain essentially stationary during electrophoresis. The choice of agarose is also dependent on the specific protein being determined, e.g. Miles Seravac Agarose is preferred for the quantitation of IgM, because Litex HSA tends to give low results.

Staining and destaining solutions. See Agarose Gel Electrophoresis.

Antisera. Rabbit antihuman sera to the specific proteins to be quantitated. Choice of antiserum is determined by its composition, specificity, avidity, antibody titre and stability. Antibodies to human proteins are best produced in rabbits because of their excellent precipitating qualities and as human pre-cipitins against serum proteins of this animal seldom occur. The use of the purified immunoglobulin fraction of antiserum is recommended. It is advantageous to know the antibody titre of specific antisera. The interbatch titre variation should be less than 10%, and loss of antibody activity less than 2% per year. We have found that Dakopatts A/S Denmark produce highly specific, avid, high titre, stable, well characterized antibodies.

Method

Preparation of agarose gel plate (1.0 mm in thickness). The selected agarose is boiled in 100 ml of veronal-glycine-tris buffer diluted 1:1 with distilled water. *See* Agarose Gel Electrophoresis. To pour plate.—

(*i*) A U-frame $205 \times 110 \times 1.0$ mm is lightly wetted with tap water and placed between two glass plates $205 \times 110 \times 1.5$ mm firmly pressed together by means of bulldog clips. Pouring of agarose is facilitated if the longer edges of the two plates are secured slightly staggered—approximately 5.0 mm on either side of the U-frame.

(*ii*) The mould is warmed in a 90°C oven for 2 min before running molten agarose down the side of the mould with a Pasteur pipette to form a 5 mm deep agarose gel seal at the base. This mould is returned to the 90°C oven for 2 min before pouring the antibody-containing agarose.

(*iii*) 30 ml of boiling agarose poured into a previously warmed 50 ml measuring cylinder. When the agarose has cooled to 56°C the appropriate amount of specific antiserum is added by automatic pipette. Careful mixing must follow to ensure even distribution of the antibodies throughout the gel.

(*iv*) The antibody containing agarose is poured as quickly as possible down the side of the warm mould taking care to avoid trapping air bubbles. The gel is allowed to set at room temperature for 20 min. The bulldog clips are removed and the top glass plate is cautiously eased off.

(*v*) The U-frame is gently removed and antibody free molten agarose is pipetted around the sides of the gel to secure it on the glass plate and prevent distortion of the outer rocket-shaped immunoprecipitates.

(*vi*) The gel plate is secured in the gel punching template and wells 2.5 mm in diameter are cut with the telescopic puncher. The position of the row of wells is dependent on the charge of the antigen to be quantitated. The first and last wells should be at least 2 cm in from the edge of the plate to prevent distortion of the immunoprecipitates by the higher potential gradient at the sides of the plate.

Preparation and application of samples. The pH and ionic strength of the samples should be close to that of the electrophoresis buffer. However, it is immaterial whether serum samples are diluted in buffer or sodium chloride 9 g/l. By automatic micropipette, precisely 3 μl of appropriately diluted samples, control and standards are applied to the wells immediately after they have been cut. The following details are important—

(*i*) The fluid surface in the well should be slightly concave to eliminate the risk of antigen spreading around the well. The wells must not be damaged.

(*ii*) A set of 4 to 5 serially diluted standards are best applied to the wells towards the middle of the row.

(*iii*) A separate dilution of the control sample is placed in every tenth well. The first and last wells contain the same diluted sample in order to ascertain whether there has been a drift during electrophoresis.

(*iv*) To ensure minimum diffusion of samples prior to electrophoresis the time between the first and last sample application must not exceed 10 min.

Electrophoresis. The glass plate is transferred to the electrophoretic chamber immediately after the wells are filled, contact being made between the gel plate and buffer by means of moistened Wettex strips via the agarose bridges. Extreme care must be taken when making contact with the Wettex strips as any excessive pressure on the gel plate, particularly near the wells may result in distortion of the rocket-shaped immunoprecipitates. Water cooling of the gel plate is necessary during electrophoresis. The time necessary for electrophoresis and the voltage applied is mainly dependent on the electrophoretic mobility of the antigen and its binding to antibody. Peak heights of 10–40 mm are the most satisfactory.

Staining of rocket-shaped immunoprecipitates—

(*i*) The gel is pressed for 15 min using 31 ET chromatography paper as described for agarose gel electrophoresis.

(*ii*) The plate is completely dried at 90°C before removing the 31 ET chromatography paper.

(*iii*) After washing the plate with cold tap water it is placed in Coomassie Brilliant Blue for 10 min.

(*iv*) The plate is washed again in cold tap water and then destained for approximately 10 min to remove excess dye.

(*v*) Destainer is washed from the plate with cold tap water and the plate returned to 90°C oven to dry.

Calculation of antigen concentration. Peak heights of 10–40 mm are most satisfactory for determining antigen concentrations. Immunoprecipitates of these heights closely correlate to the amount of antigen applied. Careful and critical inspection of the precipitation patterns must precede the measurement of the peaks. The shape and appearance of the immunoprecipitates formed by both standards and samples must be similar before calculation of the antigen concentration can be made from the standards. Calculation is as follows—

(*i*) The height of each standard peak is precisely measured in mm.

(*ii*) A standard curve is constructed to actual size on millimetre graph paper, plotting peak height on the ordinate against concentration on the abscissa.

(*iii*) The concentration of individual samples and controls are then read by sliding the plate, with the bottom of the wells along the abscissa, until the top of the peak tangents the calibration curve. The results are then corrected for sample dilution. Some workers prefer to place the gel plate face downwards on the graph paper to reduce parallax error.

Technical comments

Samples. Specific proteins present in serum, plasma, urine and other body fluids may be quantitated by electroimmunoassay. The reported lower limit of detection is approximately 300 μg/l by the protein staining procedure described.

Quality control. Commercial controls are available for most specific proteins. However, care must be exercised in the selection of commercial controls as their electrophoretic mobility and precipitation patterns are not always similar to the samples being determined. A serum pool such as that used for agarose gel electrophoresis is preferable.

Gel thickness of 1 mm is recommended. The risk of irregular migration of the precipitation front increases with gel thickness. Uniform field strength over the entire gel is critical in electroimmunoassay for reliable quantitation.

Antiserum concentration in gel must be evaluated for each specific protein to be quantitated. Peak heights between 10 and 40 mm give the best reproducibility. In general the lowest antiserum concentration possible should be used to achieve this peak height, whilst ensuring that immunoprecipitation has gone to completion and the rocket-shaped immunoprecipitates are neither too faint nor too marked. A standard curve may be adequately constructed from 4 serial dilutions of a reference sample. The slope of the standard curve is important and is determined by (a) concentration of antisera used, and (b) concentration range of the reference samples.

Storage of gel. An antibody-containing gel provided it is well sealed within its mould to avoid dehydration or microbial contamination, may be stored at 4°C for one week before use.

Direct reading standard curve permits determination of unknown samples in g/l and may be produced as follows—

(*i*) Ascertain by experiment the highest concentration of antigen to give a peak height of 40 mm for a given amount of specific antiserum, to establish the working range.

(*ii*) Calculate appropriate dilution for the unknown samples to fit within the working range of the plate.

(*iii*) Dilute reference sample by a suitable factor to give a top standard value equal to that of the highest antigen concentration tolerated.

$$\text{This dilution factor} = \frac{\text{Concentration of reference sample} \times \text{dilution of unknown}}{\text{Highest antigen concentration tolerated}}$$

e.g.

Concentration of reference sample	$= 2.0$ g/l
Dilution of unknown sample	$= \times 10$
Highest antigen concentration tolerated	$= 4.0$ g/l
Suitable dilution factor	$= \dfrac{2.0 \times 10}{4.0} = 5$

Carbamylation. Antigens with a charge similar to that of the antibodies will often produce immunoprecipitin lines unsuitable for quantitation. Slow migrating proteins such as IgG and IgM form anodic-cathodic precipitates the sum of which must be used for quantitation. Partial conversion of the amino groups of the antigen to carbamylamino groups with cyanate will increase the anodic mobility of the protein. This will result in the production of well defined immunoprecipitates. One volume of sample is mixed with one volume of 2 M potassium cyanate and incubated at 37°C for 2 h. Alternatively the mixture may be incubated at 45°C for 30 min. The same degree of carbamylation may be obtained by standing at room temperature overnight. The reaction is retarded by making appropriate dilution with saline or buffer after which the sample is ready for application in the well. It is essential that the standard and samples are treated the same to ensure that comparable carbamylation has been obtained, to give similar immunoprecipitate heights.

Variation in immunoprecipitate appearance may be due to following.—
(*i*) Differences in the precipitability of the different antigen-antibody complexes.—(*a*) Sharpness of the immunoprecipitate tip varies with the electrophoretic mobility of the protein and the rate of development of the precipitate. (b) Small antigen molecules with mobilities very close to that of the corresponding antibodies will not give evaluable peaks even after prolonged electrophoresis. (c) Immunoglobulins such as IgG and IgM which are electrophoretically and antigenically heterogeneous present analytical problems when quantitated by electroimmunoassay due to their production of anodic and cathodic precipitates. The enclosed area gives a measure of the antigen content, assuming that the standards and samples have the same electrophoretic and antigenic heterogeneity. Carbamylation prior to quantitation of such proteins alters their charge so that only an anodic precipitate is formed. (d) The antigenic heterogeneity of immunoglobulins and the varying degree of antigenic specificity of commercial antisera, suggest that immunochemical estimations of immunoglobulins are less reliable than those of other proteins. This is particularly true for the restricted antigenic determinants of monoclonal immunoglobulins. (e) Monoclonal immunoglobulins do not precipitate normally by electroimmunoassay and will often produce faintly stained, bulging precipitates.
(*ii*) Experimental conditions.—

	Appearance	Technical Cause
(a)	Atypical peaks due to antigen enrichment on surface of gel.	Overflow of well.
(b)	Abnormally narrow precipitin lines and erroneously reduced height.	Incomplete filling of well.
(c)	Short, broad, double contoured precipitates, particularly with antigen of low charge and concentration.	Rapid migration from well.
(d)	Double contoured precipitates.	Uneven temperature in gel due to excessive thickness.

Appearance	Technical Cause
(e) Uneven peak heights due to differences in speed of antigen migration.	Differences in ionic strength between top and bottom layers of gel due to evaporation.
(f) Blasted rockets, *i.e.* immunoprecipitin lines do not extend down to well.	Potential gradient too high with inadequate electrophoresis time.
(g) Oblique rockets.	Poor contact between wick and gel, or unequal thickness of gel, or electrophoresis apparatus not placed horizontally.
(h) More than one precipitin peak.	Antiserum contains antibodies against more than one protein, or partial immunochemical identity and/or electrophoretic heterogeneity of proteins, or current interrupted before end of electrophoresis.

Quantitation of specific proteins

Analytical requirements for the quantitation of proteins by electroimmunoassay vary for each specific protein. The specifications for some specific protein

Table 2.4. Specifications for some specific protein determinations

	IgG	IgA	IgM	Albumin	Transferrin
Agarose	Litex HSA	Litex HSA	Miles Seravac	Litex HSA	Litex HSA
Dako antisera per 30 ml of agarose (μl)	350	250	200	250	100
Dilution of sample	$\times 40$	$\times 10$	$\times 10$	$\times 100$	$\times 20$
Voltage (V)	200	200	150	200	200
Time (h)	2	$2\frac{1}{2}$	2	2	2
Working range (g/l)	1–16	0.2–2.8	0.2–2.2	2–52	0.2–3.4

analyses are listed in Table 2.4. The conditions listed for IgA were used to obtain the results seen in Fig. 2.7.

The quantitation of immunoglobulins presents problems in standardization due to differences in (a) source of antibody; (b) heterogeneity in antigen content of reference and test samples; (c) techniques used, *i.e.* electroimmunoassay, single radial immunodiffusion or automated immunoprecipitation. See review by Reimer & Maddison (1976).

It is important that each laboratory establishes its own reference values for the specific proteins being quantitated. As a guide, the adult reference values for serum immunoglobulins from our own protein laboratory are: IgG 7.0–13·0 g/l, IgA 0.8—3.5 g/l, IgM 0.6–2.0 g/l.

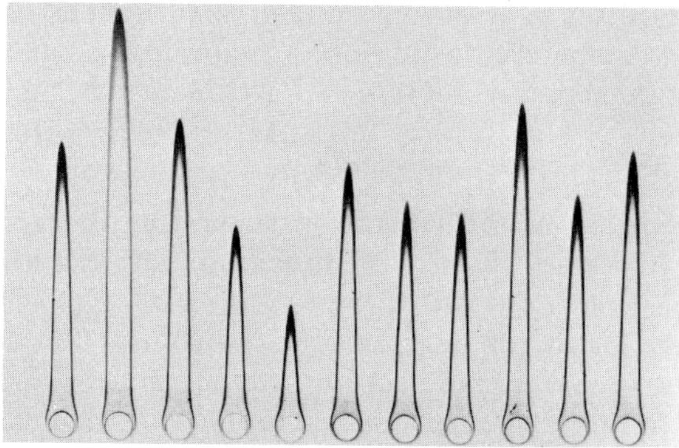

Figure 2.7. Rocket-shaped immunoprecipitates by electroimmunoassay.

Single radial immunodiffusion (Mancini)

Single radial immunodiffusion (Mancini, Carbonara & Heremans, 1965) provides an alternative means for the quantitation of specific proteins such as serum immunoglobulins and complement. Antigen is allowed to diffuse radially into agarose gel containing monospecific antiserum. The area of the precipitin ring formed at equivalence of antigen to antibody is proportional to the concentration of the antigen. A wide range of single radial immunodiffusion plates (SRID) are available from several commercial sources. It is important that the manufacturer's directions are strictly observed.

Choice of single radial immunodiffusion plate
   (*i*) Some manufacturers prepare immunodiffusion plates with different concentration ranges, since adequate precision and accuracy cannot be achieved on the same plate for an infinite range of antigen concentrations. It is therefore necessary to choose an immunodiffusion plate with the appropriate working range for the antigen being quantitated.
  (*ii*) The thickness of the gel must be uniform throughout the entire plate, and the cylindrical wells must be cleanly and uniformly cut, and positioned a suitable distance from each other, to avoid interactions with adjacent samples.
 (*iii*) The antibody contained within the gel must be of uniform concentration and be specific to the antigen being quantitated. Immunoglobulins differ in their antigenic determinants and will reflect this heterogeneous property in their reaction with specific antisera. Provided antiserum is prepared against normal polyclonal immunoglobulins and that normal immunoglobulins are used as standard antigens for calibration purposes, polyclonal immunoglobulins may be adequately quantitated.
  (*iv*) There should be only minimal interbatch, interlot variation in the quality of single radial immunodiffusion plates. The conscientious use of standards will compensate for these minor variations.
   (*v*) The condition of the plate after transportation and storage at 4–6°C is a major consideration. Excessive condensation and the presence of water in

the wells will result in erroneous antigen quantitations. It is essential that the wells are dry before the addition of samples and standards.

(*vi*) The limit of detection of SRID is approximately 0.5 μg of antigen.

Use of single radial immunodiffusion plate

(*i*) Precise application of the volume of standards, controls and unknown samples as directed by the manufacturer is essential for accurate quantitation.

(*ii*) A set of three standards is generally adequate for the construction of a calibration curve. Some manufacturers actually state where, under standard conditions, the linear plot extrapolated to zero antigen concentration should intercept the ordinate. This forms a reference point for the location of the calibration curve.

(*iii*) An appropriate control sample, either commercial or a pooled serum, together with a set of standards should be applied to each plate when determining the antigen concentration of unknown samples. However, if more than one plate is required for the number of unknown samples to be quantitated, one set of standards is adequate, provided that the plates are of the same lot and batch number and a control sample is placed on each plate.

(*iv*) Diffusion time is dependent on (a) absolute quantity of antigen applied; (b) diffusion characteristics of the antigen; (c) temperature (increase reduces the time for complete diffusion, without affecting the final size of the precipitin ring). Incubation of plates at ambient temperature is usually satisfactory for quantitation. At the expense of some loss of accuracy and sensitivity, high antigen concentrations may be determined within 4–24h depending on the specific antigen under investigation. This is the Fahey technique whereby the logarithm of the antigen concentration is plotted against the diameter of the precipitin ring. The shorter the diffusion time before reading the results, the more curvilinear the standard curve will be. Although diffusion time is longer, the Mancini technique results in more precise antigen measurements. When the antigen–antibody reaction is allowed to go to completion, the area enclosed by the precipitin ring is linearly proportional to the amount of antigen applied and to the reciprocal of the antibody concentration in the gel. The minimum diffusion time required for the quantitation of proteins such as IgG, IgA, C3 and C4 by the Mancini technique is 50 h whilst that for IgM is 80 h.

(*v*) After an appropriate diffusion time the diameters of the precipitin rings are read to the nearest 0.1 mm. This is facilitated by measuring the precipitin diameters with a graduated eye-piece, against a dark background with the light entering at right angles.

(*vi*) If all the wells are not utilized on a plate they may be used on a subsequent occasion provided the plate is stored between 4–6°C. It is advisable to apply a new set of standards.

Construction of standard curve

A standard curve is prepared by plotting the squared diameters of the three standard precipitin rings on the ordinate against their respective concentrations along the abscissa, on linear graph paper. Unknown sample values are determined by taking the intercepts of their squared diameters from the calibration curve and applying any required dilution factor. N.B. The precipitin rings must be circular for reliable quantitation. Distorted precipitin rings must be rejected. A curve which is convex upwards, suggests incomplete diffusion of the higher antigen concentrations, whilst a concave curve betokens technical error.

Standards

Standard immunoglobulin preparations used should be calibrated against World Health Organisation (WHO) Immunoglobulin Standards.

Sources of error
Antigen properties. The presence of protein complexes, polymers, and subunits will affect the quantitation of antigen concentration. Depending on the specificity of the antiserum, solutions containing related antigens will give more than one precipitin ring. In the case of antigenically heterogeneous immunoglobulins, when a broad spectrum polyclonal specific antiserum is used, only one precipitin ring will be visualized. Double precipitin rings may be seen in some instances, *e.g.* the presence of 7s and 11s IgA in the sample or the presence of normal polyclonal immunoglobulin with a monoclonal immunoglobulin. There may be other problems.—

(*i*) Protein complexes, *e.g.* Haptoglobin-haemoglobin complexes will be underestimated by single radial immunodiffusion.

(*ii*) Polymers, *e.g.* polymeric forms of IgA and IgM will also be quantitatively underestimated. Secretory 11S IgA is known to diffuse to only 70% of the extent of an equivalent weight of 7S IgA.

(*iii*) Subunits, *e.g.* low molecular weight moieties such as 7S IgM are overestimated by single radial immunodiffusion.

(*iv*) Monoclonal immunoglobulins are usually overestimated by a factor which is dependent on the degree of antigenic difference between the spectrum of normal and individual monoclonal immunoglobulin.

(*v*) Excessive antigen concentration will inhibit the formation of a visible precipitate. This may cause erroneous low levels to be reported.

(*vi*) Occasionally, IgM polymers, or cryoglobulins will not diffuse into the agarose plate thereby yielding low or absent values.

(*vii*) Rheumatoid factor may cause precipitation around the well due to interaction with the antibody in the gel, thus invalidating the antigen quantitation.

Experimental conditions.

(*i*) Unequal volumes of antigen solutions in wells and inadequate filling of wells. Overloading of wells. Spillage of antigen around outside of well. Use of plate containing either water in the wells or excessive condensation. Damaged wells, *e.g.* a cut in the agar will produce a distorted precipitin ring.

(*ii*) Analysis of unknown and standard samples after different diffusion times. Inaccurate reading of the precipitin rings.

(*iii*) Incorrect construction of standard curve. Use of manufacturers calibration tables without the rigid use of control samples and standardized conditions.

(*iv*) Denaturation of reference and unknown samples.

Preparation of immunodiffusion plate

Whilst commercially made single radial immunodiffusion plates are readily available, individual laboratories may choose to prepare their own plates. A radial immunodiffusion plate is prepared as for electroimmunoassay. It is preferable to use the plate without delay, although it may be stored as described previously. *See* Electroimmunoassay. The appropriate concentration of antiserum is ascertained by experiment, being determined by the antigen concentration range, sensitivity, and required precision.

Uniform, cylindrical wells 2.5 mm in diameter are cleanly punched at a suitable distance, approximately 15 mm from each other. A telescopic gel puncher, and punching template facilitate this procedure.

Application of samples. Precise volumes *e.g.* 5 μl of unknown and reference samples are applied to the wells. The plates are placed in a humidifier at room temperature and left in a horizontal position until diffusion of the antigen is complete.

Determination of antigen concentration. Calculation of the unknown antigen concentrations is determined as for commercial radial immunodiffusion plates.

Single radial immunodiffusion and electroimmunoassay comparison

Both methods are capable of producing similar accuracy and precision and are of equal sensitivity. They are excellent in routine quantitative clinical work although Laurell points out that single radial immunodiffusion is the method of choice for quantitating proteins with molecular weights below 40 000. Results are obtained faster by electroimmunoassay which can be an advantage in routine clinical work, but less equipment is required for single radialimmunodiffusion. A recent study by Whicher et al (1978) showed that immunodiffusion gave good immunoglobulin quantitation, while electroimmunoassay was worse than expected. This study also showed that measurement of IgA gave different results by the two methods.

Quantitation of monoclonal immunoglobulins

It is not possible to obtain an absolute value for a monoclonal immunoglobulin when the equivalence of the antigen-antibody reaction is compared with a set of normal serum standards. The only standard which can validly be used to quantitate a monoclonal immunoglobulin is that same monoclonal immunoglobulin in a purified form. Monoclonal immunoglobulins do not always precipitate normally by electroimmunoassay and single radial immunodiffusion tends to overestimate the concentration of monoclonal immunoglobulins by a factor dependent on the degree of antigenic difference between the spectrum of normal and individual monoclonal immunoglobulin.

Results obtained serially by single radial immunodiffusion using a set of normal serum standards will yield a useful index of changes in concentration of the monoclonal immunoglobulin. In conjunction with zone electrophoresis it is of value in assessing (a) the progression of the disease and (b) the patient's response to therapy.

An alternative method for quantitating monoclonal immunoglobulins is by quantitative electrophoresis. This procedure has limitations because of the differential uptake of dye by proteins and the imprecision of densitometry. Recently a procedure has been described using the dye Procion Brilliant Blue R.S. The protein fractions which have been separated on cellulose acetate are stained and eluted prior to quantitation. Problems of differential dye uptake seem to be eliminated by the use of Procion Brilliant Blue R.S., and quantitative results have shown good agreement with the micro-Kjeldahl technique. For details, see Kohn (1976).

QUALITATIVE IMMUNOELECTROPHORESIS

Immunoelectrophoresis is a two step procedure in which proteins are characterized by their electrophoretic and immunological properties.

The proteins are first separated in agarose gel by electrophoresis and subsequently identified with appropriate antisera by a process of diffusion.

Immunoelectrophoresis provides a means by which abnormal discrete bands visualized on zone electrophoresis are characterized.

Equipment
See Equipment for Protein Analyses.

Direct current power supply—Electrophoretic chamber—Wettex strips $200 \times 20 \times 3$ mm—Levelling table—Magnetic stirrer hot plate—Glass plate $205 \times 110 \times 1.5$ mm divided into eight 25 mm sections, the centre of each being marked with a diamond pen—Shandon cutter—Beakers for dispensing agarose: 50 ml; 200 ml—Hamilton syringe—50 μl automatic pipette—Stitch-cutter—19 gauge flat bevelled hypodermic needle—Weight approximately 2 kg for pressing—31 ET chromatography paper—Humidifier at room temperature—Oven at 90°C.

Reagents
Electrophoretic buffer. Tris-veronal-sodium veronal buffer (0.1 M, pH 8.8). *See* Agarose Gel Electrophoresis.The following two buffers give equivalent results.—
(*i*) Veronal-glycine-tris buffer, pH 8.8, ionic strength 0.08. *See* Electroimmunoassay.
(*ii*) Sodium-acetate-sodium veronal buffer pH 8.2, ionic strength 0.10, prepared from veronal-sodium 8.14 g, sodium acetate (anhydrous) 6.47 g, 0.1 M HCl 90 ml, made up to 1 litre with distilled water. The buffer is diluted 1 : 1 with distilled water before use.

Agarose. Suitable sources are Miles Seravac 10 g/l, BDH 10 g/l or Litex LSA 20 g/l. *See* Agarose Gel Electrophoresis.

Staining and destaining solutions. See Agarose Gel Electrophoresis.

Antisera. Rabbit antihuman serum to (a) whole serum; (b) IgG, IgA, IgM,

IgD, IgE (specific for heavy chains); (c) kappa and lambda light chains; (d) other specific proteins.

The best antisera for detecting monoclonal immunoglobulins detect any κ or λ monoclonal light chains whether free or immunoglobulin bound; they enable the monoclonal nature of a suspected paraprotein to be verified.

Method

Preparation of agarose gel plate (approximately 1.0 mm in thickness). Preparation of the plate is similar to that for Agarose Gel Electrophoresis. N.B. The slit former is NOT used. After the agarose has gelled—approximately 10 min, the plate is placed in a humidifier for 10 min for the gel to set, thus allowing

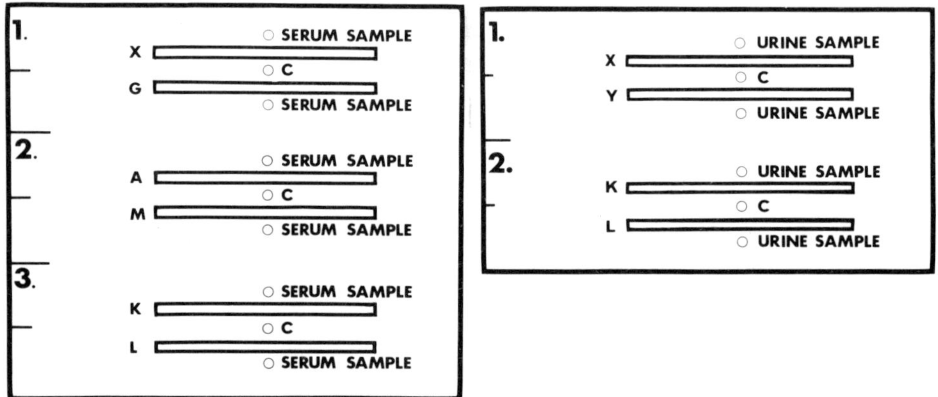

Figure 2.8 *a, b.* Scheme for identification by immunoelectrophoresis of abnormal discrete bands visualized on serum or urine protein electrophoresis.

the wells to be cut cleanly. The Shandon cutter is used to cut wells approximately 0.5 mm in diameter. These are cleared by suction with a 19 gauge flat bevelled hypodermic needle connected to a vacuum water pump.

Application of samples. With a Hamilton syringe, 1 μl of control serum is applied in the centre well of each 25 mm section, and 1 μl of patient's serum or concentrated urine is applied to the wells on either side. The samples should be applied as soon as the wells are cut to forestall gel buffer collecting in the wells. The sample in the well should be level with the gel surface for optimum electrophoresis, and wells must not be damaged as this will result in poor quality electrophoresis. Figs. 2.8a, 2.8b show suggested sample placings.

Separation of proteins by electrophoresis requires a potential gradient of 20 V/cm and a water-cooling temperature of 10–15°C as for Agarose Gel Electrophoresis. Electrophoresis should stop when the albumin front is approximately 20 mm from the anodal Wettex strip, *i.e.* after about 45 min.

Addition of specific antisera. When electrophoresis is completed the plate is taken from the electrophoretic chamber and placed in the humidifier for 10 min. Although not essential, this step facilitates the cutting of well defined troughs. These equidistant from the wells, are cut at appropriate positions with the Shandon cutter, and the gel strips carefully removed with a stitch cutter. To avoid distortion of the precipitin arcs it is of the utmost importance that the troughs are undamaged.

Approximately 50 μl of the appropriate specific antiserum is delivered to each trough by automatic pipette; the antiserum in the trough should be level with the gel surface. The plate is returned to the humidifier at an even temperature for 18–24 h or longer during which time the antibodies diffuse into the gel and react with their specific antigens resulting in white precipitin arcs.

Staining of immunoprecipitates. The gel is pressed for 3–4 h using 31 ET chromatography paper as for Agarose Gel Electrophoresis. Pressing the gel removes unreacted protein and gives a thin film. This is preferable to removing the unreacted protein by washing in several changes of saline or buffer for 48 h. The plate is completely dried at 90°C before removing the chromatography paper. After washing the plate with cold tap water it is placed in Coomassie Brilliant Blue for 5 min, washed again in cold tap water and then destained for approximately 15 min to remove excess dye. Destainer is washed from the plate with cold tap water, and the plate is placed in 90°C oven to dry. Before photographing, the plate is labelled with Indian ink.

Technical comments
Glass plates may be replaced by microscope slides secured in a tray, into which the molten agarose is poured; individual slides are cut free prior to staining.

Samples. Serum, plasma, or urine may be used. The sample is routinely applied undiluted, however, in some instances when excessive amounts of protein are present, typing is facilitated by dilution. Urine is concentrated to give approximately 25 g protein/l; an early morning urine sample is adequate and should be analysed as fresh as possible. (*See* Chapter 6, Urine Protein Electrophoresis). Ideally, immunoelectrophoresis of the patient's serum and urine samples should be carried out on the same plate, to permit direct comparison of reactions.

Quality control. The pooled serum with which each patient's serum is compared consists of at least seven normal sera. The albumin is tagged by adding 50 μl of serum protein diluent as for Agarose Gel Electrophoresis, or a pinch of Bromphenol Blue.

Treatment with 2-mercaptoethanol reduces disulphide bonds and facilitates light chain typing of monoclonal IgM. One drop of mercaptoethanol is added to 0.5 ml of patient serum and vortexed continuously for 10 min to avoid gelling prior to immunoelectrophoresis.

Relative concentration of antigen and antibody should approach optimum proportions for immunoprecipitation.

Interpretation of qualitative immunoelectrophoresis
Antigens are identified by comparing the precipitin arc of each test sample in configuration and mobility with the control. In complex protein mixtures, antigen-antibody interactions of double immunodiffusion type may be observed. A monoclonal immunoglobulin manifests itself by distortion of the precipitin arc. To characterize a monoclonal immunoglobulin the abnormal bowing and/or

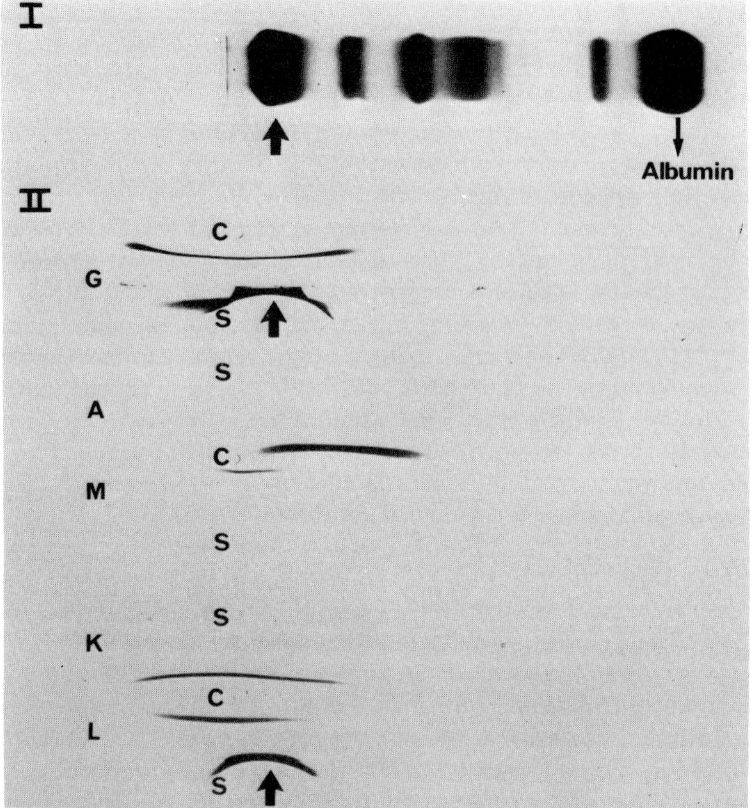

Figure 2.9. I. Abnormal discrete band (heavy arrow) on the serum protein electrophoretogram. II. Abnormal bowing and thickening of IgG and lambda arcs, (arrows), correspond in position to the abnormal band in I. IgA and IgM arcs of the test sample are not visible due to associated immunoparesis.

G = antiIgG	A = antiIgA	M = antiIgM
K = antikappa	L = antilambda	S = serum sample wells
C = control serum wells		

thickening of the heavy chain immunoglobulin component must not only correspond in position to the abnormal configuration of the light chain component, either kappa or lambda, but also to the discrete band visualized on zone electrophoresis (Fig. 2.9). There are cases in which more than one monoclonal immunoglobulin or component thereof are encountered, and others with monoclonal light chains only.

Crossed immunoelectrophoresis (Laurell)

Crossed immunoelectrophoresis is a two-step procedure in which proteins may be identified according to their electrophoretic and immunochemical properties. The proteins are first separated in antibody-free agarose gel by electrophoresis. The protein fractions to be identified are then electrophoresed perpendicularly into gel containing specific antibody. Crossed immunoelectrophoresis has high resolution and is an effective tool even for analysing complex antigen-antibody systems. In patients with renal disease, the test has received widest application in assessing complement activation by the measurement of C3 breakdown products and in the detection of C3 nephritic factor (C3NeF). *See* Chapter 3.

Equipment
See Equipment for Protein Analyses.

Direct current power supply—Electrophoretic chambers as in (a) Agarose gel Electrophoresis, and (b) Electroimmunoassay—Wettex strips $200 \times 20 \times 3$ mm, and for 2nd dimension electrophoresis $200 \times 25 \times 3$ mm—Levelling table—Magnetic stirrer hot plate—Three glass plates, $205 \times 110 \times 1.5$ mm—One U-frame, $205 \times 110 \times 1.0$ mm—Slit former, rectangular teeth, 0.5 mm—Beakers: 50 ml; 200 ml—50 ml fine-lipped measuring cylinder—$3 \mu l$ automatic pipette—Stitch cutter—Clear plastic ruler—Dialysis tubing (optional)—Thermometer 0–$110°$C—Weight approximately 2 kg for pressing—31 ET chromatography paper—Oven at $90°$C.

Reagents
Electrophoresis buffers (a) Tris-veronal-sodium veronal buffer, 0.1 M, pH 8.8 as in Agarose Gel Electrophoresis (b) Veronal-glycine-tris buffer, pH 8.8, ionic strength 0.08 as in Electroimmunoassay.

Agarose. Miles Seravac 10 g/l. Litex HSA 15 g/l.

Antisera. Rabbit antihuman serum to the specific proteins to be investigated as in Qualitative Immunoelectrophoresis.

Fixing, staining, destaining solutions as in Agarose Gel Electrophoresis.

Method
Preparation of antibody-free agarose gel plate as in Agarose Gel Electrophoresis.

Preparation and application of serum samples as in Agarose Gel Electrophoresis. It is recommended that both tests and control samples are applied to duplicate wells to ensure sufficient sample-containing gel for electrophoresis in the second dimension. This also acts as a reference to facilitate interpretation.

Separation of proteins in the first dimension by electrophoresis as in Agarose Gel Electrophoresis using Wettex wicks $200 \times 20 \times 3$ mm.

Preparation of antibody-containing agarose gel plate as in Electroimmunoassay. It is convenient to prepare the antibody-containing gel plate whilst the proteins are being separated in the first dimension. Litex HSA Agarose—15 g/l is generally used. Add antisera versus specific protein or proteins to be identified and if desired versus proteins of known mobility to act as markers and help interpretation.

Application of gel strip to antibody-containing agarose plate. Two minutes before completion of electrophoresis in the first dimension, the U-frame is gently removed from the antibody-containing gel plate. By means of a stitch-cutter and ruler a straight line is cut along the gel plate, approximately 30 mm from the base. The gel is carefully parted by running a finger gently between the cut portions. When the first dimension electrophoresis is completed, the gel plate is removed from the electrophoretic chamber. Uniform cuts are made in the mid-section of the agarose gel for both test and control samples using the stitch cutter and ruler. The strips of agarose should be 2–5 mm in width and of appropriate length to contain the proteins to be identified. Using the stitch cutter or scalpel blade, the agarose strips are carefully placed alongside each other on the antibody-containing gel. Avoid trapping of air bubbles or excessive handling. The lower portion of the parted agarose is gently and evenly pushed up to make good contact between the upper portion of antibody containing gel, the inserted agarose strips and the lower portion of antibody containing gel.

Fixing and staining of the first dimension plate as in Agarose Gel Electrophoresis provides a reference for interpretation of the second dimension patterns.

Electrophoresis in the second dimension. The antibody-containing gel plate is placed in the electrophoretic chamber, as for Electroimmunoassay. Contact is made between the gel plate and the buffer by means of moistened $200 \times 25 \times 3$ mm Wettex via the agarose bridges. Extreme care must be taken when making contact with the Wettex strips as excessive pressure may distort immunoprecipitation. The use of dialysis tubing is optional. Water cooling is necessary during electrophoresis. The potential gradient and time are dependent on the electrophoretic mobility of the specific antigens under investigation; 15 V/cm for 1–2 h are usually satisfactory.

Staining of the immunoprecipitates as in Electroimmunoassay.

Technical comments
Samples of serum, plasma or urine may be used.

Optimal antiserum concentration in gel is ascertained by experiment. The width of the agarose strip and the amount of protein it contains will affect the height of the peaks. Peak heights between 10–30 mm give a high resolution and facilitate evaluation.

Sources of error.
(*i*) Excessively wide agarose strips may cause electrophoretic irregularities.
(*ii*) A thin sharp blade will minimize squeezing liquid from the gel.
(*iii*) Equal size of control and test agarose strips allows direct comparison of the precipitation peaks, thus providing a semiquantitative measure.
(*iv*) The agarose strips must be transferred to the second dimension plate with extreme care; the gel must not be stretched and there should be minimal expression of fluid in the glass-gel interface to avoid distortion of the immunoprecipitates.
(*v*) The agarose strips must be positioned perpendicular to the gel surface on the second dimension plate to avoid double or oblique peaks.
(*vi*) Inadequate cooling of the gel produces poorly defined immunoprecipitin peaks and/or spurring.
(*vii*) Antigen excess results in faint immunoprecipitation while antibody excess produces very dense immunoprecipitation.
(*viii*) The quality of the second dimension pattern depends on the quality of the first dimension electrophoresis.

Quantitation by crossed immunoelectrophoresis. Laurell's method for crossed immunoelectrophoresis is semiquantitative—only part of the original sample is examined in the second dimension. However, Clarke and Freeman (1968) have modified the technique for quantitation. A lower potential gradient is used and the entire sample is run in the second dimension.

CRYOPROTEINS

Plasma proteins, normally soluble below 37°C, which may form insoluble precipitates in the cold are known as cryoproteins. The temperature at which cold precipitation occurs is influenced by a number of factors including the concentration of cryoprecipitable protein present. Cryoproteins precipitating above 21°C tend to produce clinical symptoms. The presence of cryoproteins in man often indicates an active immunological process, *e.g.* circulating immune complexes or proliferative disorders of the immune system. Their detection may be useful in assessing the pathogenesis of some clinical syndromes. Frequently they are associated with renal impairment usually due to glomerular lesions.

Cryoproteins may be classified according to their immunochemical properties into—(i) cryo-monoclonal immunoglobulin; (ii) cryo-polyclonal immunoglobulin; (iii) cryofibrinogen; (iv) mixed cryoproteins. These mixed cryoproteins may occur as (a) monoclonal immunoglobulin component possessing antibody activity to polyclonal IgG; (b) monoclonal immunoglobulin component plus cryofibrinogen; (c) one or more classes of polyclonal immunoglobulin and sometimes a non-immunoglobulin component such as complement.

The IgM-IgG rheumatoid factor is the most frequently encountered mixed cryoprotein. The IgM may be either polyclonal or monoclonal, in which case it is nearly always of kappa type, whereas the IgG antigen is always polyclonal.

Procedure for the investigation of cryoproteins
Samples. Both serum and plasma samples are required for cryoprotein screening; the plasma sample should be collected in EDTA or oxalate not heparin because it forms a cold-precipitable complex with fibrinogen and cold-insoluble globulin in normal plasma. Ideally, blood should be collected and separated in a room maintained at 37°C. Optimally the patient, preferably fasting is kept in a 37°C room for 20 min. All equipment is also kept at 37°C, including centrifuge, 20 ml syringe, collecting tubes, Pasteur pipettes and plastic serology tubes 10 × 75 mm. Blood is drawn from the patient and 10 ml is delivered into a plain tube to clot and 10 ml into a tube containing EDTA. After centrifugation, serum and plasma samples are transferred in equal aliquots to serology tubes. Samples are best preserved with sodium azide 1 g/l.

Detection of cryoproteins. A serum and plasma sample are placed at 4°C or other desired temperature, whilst control serum and plasma samples are maintained at 37°C. The test serum and plasma samples are checked for cryoprecipitation for four days. Monoclonal cryoglobulins and cryofibrinogen tend to precipitate at 4°C after 3–18 h whilst mixed cryoglobulins may not precipitate before 72 h. The appearance of a cryoprecipitate may be floccular, gelatinous or crystalline. Any precipitate observed at 4°C must be related to the appearance of the 37°C sample. If equivalent precipitation occur in 4°C and 37°C samples, it is unlikely that a cryoprotein is present, although subsequent solution at 37°C with persistent precipitate at 4°C indicates the presence of a cryoprotein.

Identification of cryoprecipitate. Cryoprecipitates may be characterized immunoelectrophoretically as follows—

(*i*) Centrifuge the sample for 10 min at 600 *g* and 4°C. Transfer supernatant to serology tube and label. Add 0.5 ml of sodium chloride 9 g/l previously cooled to 4°C to the cryoprecipitate. Mix. Add an additional 4.0 ml of cooled sodium chloride 9 g/l to the tube and centrifuge for 10 min at 600 *g*. Repeat three more times, ensuring that the fourth washing is kept.

(*ii*) For immunoelectrophoresis, the washed cryoprecipitate is redissolved at 37°C in sodium chloride 9 g/l, the volume of which is dependent on the amount of washed precipitate, to give an adequate antigen concentration for immunoelectrophoresis. This is then performed on the dissolved cryoprotein and the fourth washing, using antiserum to the specific proteins anticipated in the cryoprecipitate. The fourth washing is used to establish thorough washing of the cryoprecipitate. *See* Qualitative Immunoelectrophoresis for details.

Quantitation of cryoprotein. The amount of cryoprotein may be measured either by using the cryocrit method, which is similar to determining a haematocrit, or by quantitation using the biuret method as described by Lowry et al (1951), though this method presents standardization problems, because of differences in protein colour equivalence and non-linearity.

Significance of cryoproteins

Cryoproteins have been reported mainly in immunoproliferative and auto-immune diseases. Mixed cryoproteins are commonly thought to be immune complexes such as may occur in acute vasculitis. Cryoproteins are often detected without any associated disease.

Cryoproteins in renal disease. In addition to a syndrome associated with arthralgia, purpura and rapidly progressive glomerulonephritis, cryoproteins are associated with immune complex-mediated glomerulonephritis. Where the nature of the antigenic stimulus is known, as in malaria, syphilis, hepatitis B, streptococcal infection and systemic lupus erythematosus (S.L.E.), the cryoprecipitates resemble deposits identified in the kidney. In S.L.E., cryoprecipitates are most common in patients with active disease, renal involvement and reduced serum complement. The highest incidence of cryoproteinaemia has been found in acute poststreptococcal glomerulonephritis (100%) with a lower incidence (50%) in membranous and membranoproliferative glomerulonephritis (McIntosh et al, 1975). The cryoproteins in renal disease are associated with progression of the glomerulonephritis, while their disappearance from the serum signifies clinical improvement or impending end-stage renal disease. Fibrinogen in the cryoprecipitate often indicates a rapidly progressive glomerulonephritis and a poor prognosis. In patients presenting with haematuria or proteinuria, the detection of circulating cryoproteins supports a diagnosis of immune complex glomerulopathy.

EQUIPMENT FOR PROTEIN ANALYSES

Direct current power supply
For the majority of routine electrophoretic techniques, a direct current supply capable of a high potential gradient is required, and the following specifications are suitable—0–300 V continuously variable; 0–500 mA maximum; four output channel with parallel connection, input power, polarity and output power controlled. Automatic cutout at 300 V.

Support bridge with cooling coil (Fig. 2.10)
For most electrophoretic techniques cold tap water 10–20°C is adequate for cooling. If required, more rigorously controlled temperature may be obtained

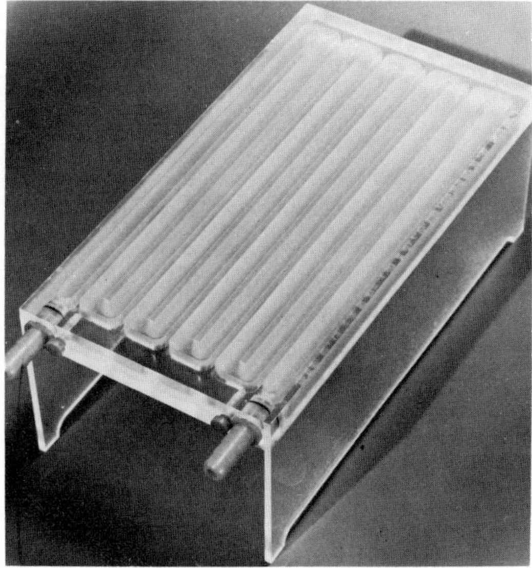

Figure 2.10. Support bridge with water cooling coil for agarose gel electrophoresis.

with a circulation thermostat. The required temperature and the flow rate of the coolant are among other things, dependent on the number of pieces of electrophoretic apparatus through which the water has to pass, the development of heat during electrophoresis and the temperature of the surroundings. Too intense cooling of the gel may result in condensation in the wells and on the surface of the gel, whilst insufficient cooling may result in increased evaporation from the gel surface and cause the gel to become more concentrated.

Buffer–gel connection
Buffer vessels should have a volume of 1 litre or more, to ensure sufficient buffering capacity, during prolonged electrophoretic runs.

Electrodes (platinum) should be embedded in a plastic groove to prevent mechanical damage. They must also be accessible so that precipitated buffer salt may be washed away, and be as far as possible from the wicks to avoid contamination by electrolytic products.

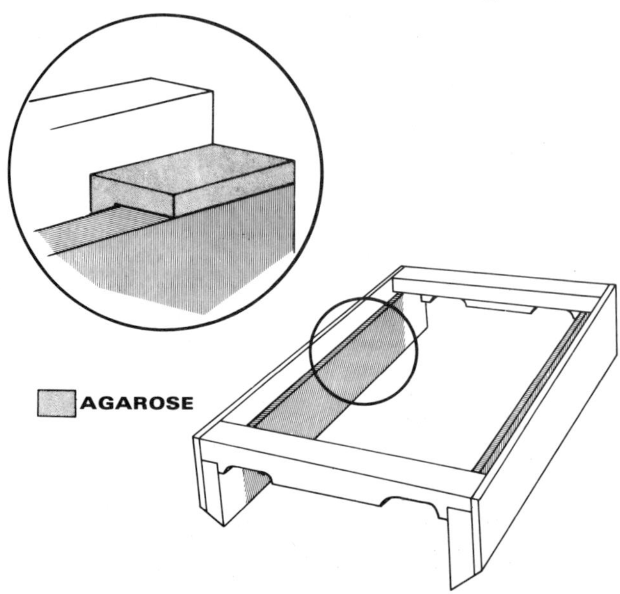

Figure 2.11. Frame for the preparation and support of agarose gel wicks. The insert shows the position of the prepared agarose gel within the frame.

Frame for gel wicks (Fig. 2.11). Agarose bridges on either side of the water cooling support, together with Wettex strips provide a suitable buffer–gel connection.

Agarose bridges 5 mm in thickness, are made with 15 g/l agarose in buffer. It is important that the agarose and buffer are the same as for electrophoresis. Hot agarose, approximately 60°C is poured into the perspex moulds of the gel frame, the bottoms of which are temporarily sealed with pressure tape. Care should be taken to ensure a good seal to prevent leakage of the molten agarose. An added precaution against leakage is to pour the mould in two steps, *i.e.* by allowing the first 10 ml of agarose to set in the bottom of the mould before completely filling it to capacity. Care must be taken to avoid air bubbles. Once the agarose has gelled within the mould, approximately 7 ml of molten agarose is run along the top of the mould to cover the top of the inner perspex plate. When the agarose has gelled the pressure tape is removed before placing the gel frame in position over the support bridge in the electrophoretic chamber. To avoid contamination of the gel wick with high molecular weight substances, clean dialysis tubing soaked in buffer may be placed between the gel wick and the Wettex strip.

Wettex strips. Absorbant household sponge, 3 mm thick soaked in buffer is used to make contact between the gel plate and agarose bridges, and cut to $200 \times 20 \times 3$ mm. The wick should allow buffer to flow at the same rate as in the agarose to prevent drying or swelling of the gel plate.

Gels

Glass plates are available in various sizes, the following dimensions are satisfactory: $205 \times 110 \times 1.5$ mm; $100 \times 100 \times 1.5$ mm.

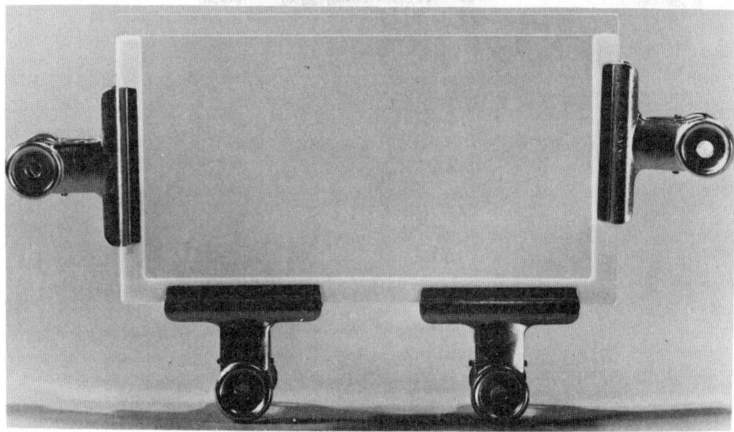

Figure 2.12. Apparatus for the preparation of agarose gels of uniform thickness.

U-Frames (Fig. 2.12) When a gel of absolute uniformity is required as in Electroimmunoassay, the agarose is allowed to set between two glass plates held apart by a U-frame 1.0–1.5 mm thick with bulldog clips to maintain a seal. Once the agarose is firmly set, in about 20 min, one plate is carefully removed together with the U-frame. The agarose plate is then ready for use.

Telescopic gel puncher provides clean cut wells. After punching out the well with a larger outer needle, gentle pressure is applied to the smaller internal needle to establish connection between the vacuum pump and the gel surface. Well cutters of varying diameters are available: 2.5 mm and 4.0 mm have been most useful.

Gel punching template (Fig. 2.13) allows wells to be punched out side by side reproducibly. This is particularly important in electroimmunoassay. The template consists of a base plate with holes, and firmly fixed above it, a narrow plexibridge with linear holes to guide the well cutter. The gel plate may be firmly fixed at any desired position under the bridge by means of metal pins inserted in the holes of the base plate.

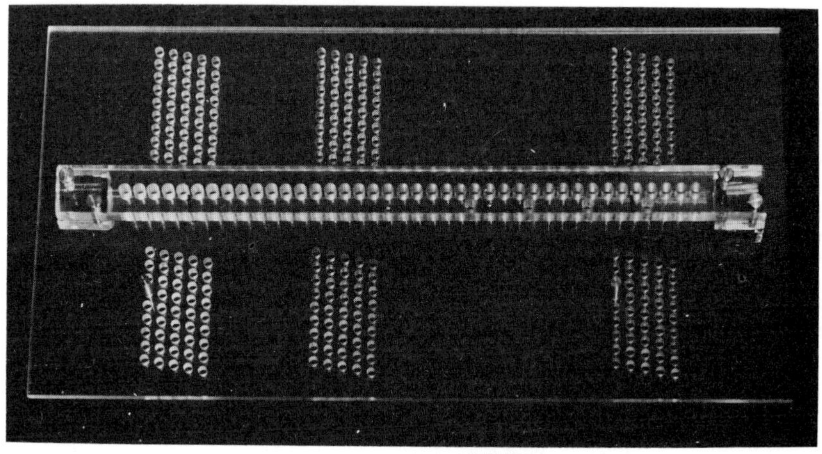

Figure 2.13. Gel punching template.

Levelling table. A horizontal table fitted with a spirit level is essential for pouring gel plates of uniform thickness for electrophoresis.

Slit Former (Fig. 2.14). This device consists of rectangular stainless steel teeth 5 mm in length and 0.4 mm thick, inserted between two perspex blocks held together with three screws. The perspex blocks stand on four umbraco

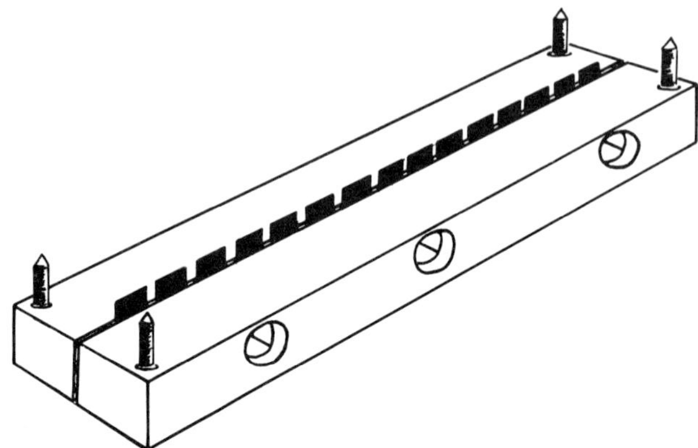

Figure 2.14. Slit-former for agarose gel electrophoresis.

screws which are adjusted on a glass plate so that the teeth are 0.1 mm from the glass. The teeth are coated with a thin film of silicone grease.

Cutter for immunoelectrophoresis. Wells of uniform diameter and troughs equidistant to these wells are required for immunoelectrophoresis. Commercial apparatus to obtain these requirements are available *e.g.* 'Shandon Cutter'. The wells are spaced three wells 0.5 mm in diameter per 25 mm section of the glass plate. The trough is cut by double blades separated by a metal spacer.

REFERENCES

Clarke H G M, Freeman T 1968 Quantitative immunoelectrophoresis of human serum proteins. Clinical Science 35: 403–413

Fahey J L, McKelvey E M 1965 Quantitative determination of serum immunoglobulins in antibody-agar plates. The Journal of Immunology 94: 84–90

Hobbs J R 1971 Immunoglobulins in clinical chemistry. In: Advances in Clinical Chemistry ed Bodansky O, Latner A L vol 14: p 219–317 Academic Press, New York and London

Kohn J 1976 Cellulose acetate electrophoresis and immunodiffusion techniques. In: Chromatographic and Electrophoretic Techniques ed Smith I vol 2: 90–137 Heinemann Medical Books, London

Laurell C-B 1972 Electroimmunoassay. Scandinavian Journal of Clinical Laboratory Investigation 29: suppl 124, 21–37

Laurell C-B, Jeppsson J-O, Tejler L 1975 Plasma Protein Analysis. ed Lane H E Millipore Corporation, Massachusetts

Lowry O H, Rosebrough N J, Farr A L, Randall R J 1951 Protein measurement with the Folin phenol reagent. The Journal of Biological Chemistry 193: 265–275

Mancini G, Carbonara A O, Heremans J F 1965 Immunochemical quantitation of antigens by single radial immunodiffusion. Immunochemistry 2: 235–254

McIntosh R M, Griswold W R, Chernack W B, Williams G, Strauss J, Kaufman D B, Koss M N, McIntosh J R, Cohen R, Weil R 1975 Cryoglobulins III. Quarterly Journal of Medicine, new series 44: 285–307

Ouchterlony Ö, Nilsson L-Å 1978 Immunodiffusion and immunoelectrophoresis. In: Handbook of Experimental Immunology ed Weir D M vol 1: ch 19, p 19.10–19.22 Blackwell, Oxford
Reimer C B, Maddison S E 1976 Standardization of human immunoglobulin quantitation: A review of current status and problems. Clinical Chemistry 22: 577–582
Whicher J T, Hunt J, Perry D E, Hobbs J R, Fifield R, Keyser J, Kohn J, Riches P, Smith A M, Thompson R A, Ward A M, White P 1978 Method-specific variations in the calibration of a new immunoglobulin standard suitable for use in nephelometric techniques. Clinical Chemistry 24: 531–535

UNCITED BIBLIOGRAPHY

Brouet J-C, Clauvel J-P, Danon F, Klein M, Seligmann M 1974 Biologic and clinical significance of cryoglobulins. The American Journal of Medicine 57: 775–788
Doumas B T 1975 Standards for total serum protein assays—A collaborative study. Clinical Chemistry 21: 1159–1166
Ganrot P O 1972 Crossed immunoelectrophoresis. Scandinavian Journal of Clinical Laboratory Investigation 29: suppl 124, 39–47
Grey H M, Kohler P F 1973 Cryoimmunoglobulins. Seminars in Haematology 10: 87–112
Johansson B G 1972 Agarose gel electrophoresis. Scandinavian Journal of Clinical Laboratory Investigation 29: suppl 124, 7–19
Reeder D J, Schaffer R 1977 Standard reference material (SRM) for total protein determinations—Bovine serum albumin. Clinical Chemistry 23: 1136
Ritzmann S E 1975 Immunoglobulin abnormalities. In: Serum Protein Abnormalities. Diagnostic and Clinical Aspects ed Ritzmann S E, Daniels J C ch 19, p 351–485 Little, Brown and Company, Boston
Rowe D S 1975 Immunoglobulins. In: Clinical Aspects of Immunology ed Gell P G H, Coombs R R A, Lachmann P J ch 12, p 285–306 Blackwell, Oxford
Spiegelberg H L 1974 Biological activities of immunoglobulins of different classes and subclasses. In: Advances in Immunology ed Dixon F J, Kunkel H G vol 19: p 259–294 Academic Press, New York and London
Stanworth D R, Turner M W 1978 Immunochemical analysis of immunoglobulins and their sub-units. In: Handbook of Experimental Immunology ed Weir D M vol 1: ch 6, p 6.1–6.102 Blackwell, Oxford
Weeke B 1973 A Manual of Quantitative Immunoelectrophoresis Methods and Applications ed Axelsen N H, Krøll J, Weeke B ch 1, 2, 3, p 15–56 Universitetsforlaget, Oslo
Williams C A, Chase M W (ed) 1971 Precipitin analysis by diffusion in gels. In: Methods in Immunology and Immunochemistry vol 3, ch 14 Academic Press, New York and London

3
Complement

A. R. McGiven

The complement system consists of at least 16 plasma components which take part in a rather complex chain of inter-related reactions triggered off in the main by antigen-antibody complexes. A good recent review is by Fothergill & Anderson (1978).

The importance of the complement system in the immunological study of patients with renal disease is twofold. The levels of serum components may indicate that complement has been consumed in the course of an immunological reaction and the identification of complement components in the renal biopsy suggests the presence of combined antigen and antibody in the kidney. The initial antigen-antibody reaction may have occurred locally in the kidney or immune complexes formed elsewhere may be carried to the kidney by the blood stream.

COMPLEMENT ACTIVATION

Classical complement pathway

All eleven components appear to be glycoproteins (Muller-Eberhard, 1975). The first stage is the conversion of C1 to its active form $C\bar{1}$ and is important because it is this step which is triggered off by immune complexes or aggregated immunoglobulins binding the C1q component. Calcium ions are required for the activation of C1r which cleaves C1s producing the active enzyme $C\bar{1}$.

The second stage is the formation of the C3 convertase C4b2a through the action of $C\bar{1}$ on the β globulins C4 and C2 in the presence of magnesium ions.

The third stage is the conversion of C3, which is also known as β1C and is the predominant complement component in plasma, to C3b. This step is the major reaction in the complement chain and is likened to the generation of fibrin in the coagulation system. A smaller product C3a is chemotactic and C3b may break down further to C3c and C3d under the influence of C3b inactivator.

The C3 convertase combines with activated C3b to act as C5 convertase and activates the remainder of the complement system to finally produce C5b6789 causing the rupture of cell membranes.

The sequence of reactions outlined briefly above would rapidly lead to exhaustion of plasma complement components were it not for various control mechanisms. In some cases a particular step is switched off because of the instability of an activated enzyme, produced as the product of the previous reaction. This is seen with activated C2. In other cases substances are present in the serum which inactivate various convertases. Inhibitors have been identified for C1 esterase and C3b.

Alternative complement pathway

In addition to the sequence of steps which form the classical pathway, an alternative pathway for the conversion of C3 to C3b has been demonstrated which does not involve C1, C2 and C4. The system is not fully characterized but is known to involve properdin (Factor P), Factor D and Factor B (C3PA).

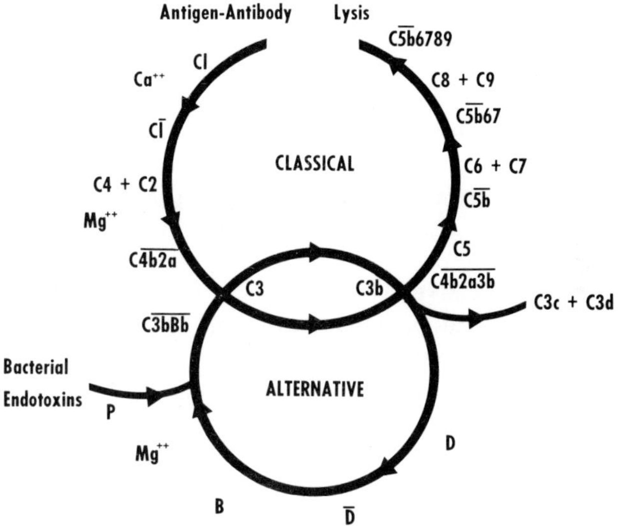

Figure 3.1. Simplified schema of classical and alternative complement activation pathways showing their inter-relationship through conversion of C3 to C3b.

Table 3.1. Physicochemical properties of complement components

Component	Molecular weight	Electrophoretic mobility	Serum concentration (μg/ml)
Classical activation pathway			
C1q	400 000	γ2	180
C1r	170 000	β	Not known
C1s	80 000	α2	120
C4	240 000	β1	250
C2	110 000	β2	30
C3	180 000	β2	1300
C5	170 000	β1	80
C6	95 000	β2	60
C7	110 000	β2	55
C8	160 000	γ1	80
C9	80 000	α	160
Alternative activation pathway			
Properdin	220 000	γ2	25
Factor D	25 000	α	Not known
Factor B	95 000	β2	240
Initiating Factor	170 000	β	Not known

The alternative pathway is activated by bacterial endotoxins, properdin, zymosan, inulin, aggregates of myeloma IgA and IgG and perhaps IgE but not IgM. C3b can stimulate further conversion of C3 to C3b in a feedback cycle. The roles of B1H and C3b inactivator are also assuming increasing importance.

The interrelationship between the classical and alternative pathways of complement activation are shown schematically in Figure 3.1. The physicochemical characteristics of the components of the classical and alternative activation pathways are given in Table 3.1.

Complement breakdown products

Estimation of cleavage products of C3, namely C3b, C3c and C3d may be useful in evaluating the significance of the serum levels of individual complement components, particularly C3. The presence of these breakdown products indicates utilization of complement regardless of whether the serum level of C3 is within or outside the normal range. A low C3 in the absence of breakdown products suggests a low rate of synthesis rather than activation by immune complexes or through the alternative pathway.

C3 nephritic factors (C3NeF)

During the investigation of patients with renal disease some patients with glomerulonephritis of the mesangiocapillary or membranoproliferative type were found to have low serum C3 levels. Study revealed that this appeared to be due, at least in part, to the generation of a C3 splitting enzyme. Incubation of the patient's serum with normal serum results in activation of C3 by the alternative pathway. Spitzer et al (1969) referred to the substance responsible as the C3 nephritic factor (C3NeF) and Scott et al (1978) have suggested that it may be an autoantibody directed against newly formed determinants on the C3 convertases C3bB and C3bBb of the alternative pathway. It belongs to the IgG class of immunoglobulins with a molecular weight of 170 000 and contains two heavy chains each of 50 000 daltons.

C3NeF is responsible for splitting C3 by stabilizing the convertase which is normally labile. Low C3 levels are also contributed to by reduced synthesis and sequestration in tissues. As C3NeF resembles initiating factor antigenically and in its molecular weight, there is some doubt as to whether these substances are different. If present in children C3NeF may persist into adult life and may be transferred across the placenta from mother to fetus (Davis et al, 1977). C3 splitting activity not necessarily due to C3NeF is also found in a significant proportion of patients with acute diffuse proliferative glomerulonephritis.

ESTIMATION OF COMPLEMENT

Collection of sample

For accurate estimations of serum complement, particularly where tests of complement function are being undertaken, care is required in the collection and processing of the blood specimen. The blood sample is withdrawn and allowed to coagulate at room temperature. The sample should not be incubated at 4°C or 37°C as is sometimes done to aid clot retraction.

After clot retraction has occurred, the serum should be withdrawn and divided into aliquots of suitable size for storage, preferably at $-70°C$. For periods of a week storage at $-20°C$ is usually satisfactory. Ideally functional haemolytic tests are performed on fresh serum.

Where breakdown products are being examined the blood sample is collected into EDTA which inactivates C1q and prevents further C3 conversion. EDTA plasma samples can also be used for the measurement of individual components.

TOTAL HAEMOLYTIC COMPLEMENT

Functional complement activity may be assessed by the ability of complement to haemolyse red blood cells which have been coated with antibodies.

Radial immunodiffusion

Total haemolytic complement can be assayed in radial immunodiffusion plates containing 1% sheep erythrocytes sensitized with haemolysin. Complement in the patient's serum permits lysis of the erythrocytes to form a clear zone around the well. A reference curve is drawn on semilog graph paper by plotting the cleared zone ring diameters of the reference sera on the linear axis and the corresponding concentrations of the standard on the logarithmic axis. Test concentrations are determined at points where the cleared zone ring diameter of the test serum intersects with the reference curve. Samples are incubated at $37°C$ for six h before reading. This test is an excellent screening procedure for the detection of impaired functional complement activity. Plates are available commercially or can be readily prepared (Lachman & Hobart, 1978).

Tube method

Estimates of haemolytic complement activity in CH50 units can be obtained from the tube technique (Mayer, 1961). One CH50 unit produces 50% haemolysis of antibody coated erythrocytes under standardized conditions. Antibody coated sheep red cells are incubated with dilutions of the patient's serum and the optical density of the supernatant is read at 541 nm which is optimal for the detection of released haemoglobin. This test is more demanding than the preceding test and is used less frequently since the advent of radial immunodiffusion techniques for the measurement of individual complement components. Strong et al (1978) have indicated inaccuracies which may occur using CH50 units and have suggested modifications.

The normal range is wide and levels of individual complement components may fall by more than 50% before changes in haemolytic complement activity are detected.

MEASUREMENT OF INDIVIDUAL COMPLEMENT COMPONENTS

The individual components of complement may be assayed functionally in a haemolytic system in which the specific component has been omitted, or measured as serum proteins by radial immunodiffusion using monospecific antisera. The former methods give a measure of functional capacity whereas the latter do not distinguish active from inactive components.

Radial immunodiffusion

The availability of suitable commercial preparations and the ease with which tests can be set up mean that most routine laboratories will prefer to use complement protein estimations. C1q, C3, C4, Factor B (C3PA) and properdin as well as some other components may be measured by this technique.

5 μl of reference samples and test sera are added to the wells and incubated for 50 h at room temperature. The diameters of the precipitin rings are measured to 0.1 mm. A reference curve is drawn on graph paper by plotting the squared diameter of the three standard precipitin rings on the ordinate against their respective concentrations along the abscissa on linear graph paper.

Less precise quantitation is obtained by the Fahey technique where the precipitin ring is measured within 24 h and the logarithm of the antigen concentration is plotted against the diameter of the precipitin ring.

Disadvantages of radial immunodiffusion measurement of complement are that it takes 24–50 h to reach an end point and during this time reaction products of complement components may appear and result in falsely high measurements. C3c(β1A), a conversion product of C3(β1C), is detected by commercial C3 antisera which have activity against β1C and β1A. The more rapidly diffusing small molecule C3c will form a ring of larger diameter than the native C3. C3c may be generated by mishandling of the specimen and by repeated freezing and thawing.

There may be some variation in reading the ring diameter by individual observers and as this measurement is then squared, any error is compounded. For this reason it may be preferable for one observer to read all reactions and plot the reference curve.

Where the diameter is near the well margin estimation of the diameter may be unsatisfactory. If the serum under test has been diluted before testing it can then be retested again without dilution.

In spite of the possible disadvantages discussed above, radial immuno-diffusion remains the method of choice for measuring complement components in routine laboratories.

See Single Radial Immunodiffusion in Chapter 2 for detailed consideration of this technique.

Electroimmunoassay (Laurell rocket technique)

Complement components can also be measured by the electrophoresis of serum into agarose gel containing monospecific antisera (Laurell, 1972). The height of the peak is compared with known standards and is a measure of the concentration of the complement component. This method is quicker and any effects from conversion of complement factors and reaction with the gel are considerably reduced.

Laboratories already employing this technique for the estimation of certain serum proteins may prefer to use it for serum complement measurements. *See* Electroimmunoassay in Chapter 2 for technical details.

Measurement of complement breakdown products

C3 and its breakdown products share at least four antigens and their distribution is shown in Table 3.2. Anti-C3 (β1C/β1A) serum reacts with native C3, C3b, C3c and may also detect C3d. As yet few monospecific antisera directed against C3 antigens are commercially available. Antiserum against the 'C'

Table 3.2. Antigenic characteristics of C3 and its breakdown products

Component	Native C3 antigen	A	C	D
Native C3	+	+	+	+
C3a		+		
C3b			+	+
C3c			+	
C3d				+

antigen of C3 will react with native C3, C3b and C3c but not with C3a or C3d. Because native C3 has β1C electrophoretic mobility and the C3c breakdown products have β1A mobility these components can be distinguished by crossed immunoelectrophoresis using the above antiserum.

Specimen

A blood sample is collected into EDTA and the plasma separated by centrifugation within 30 min if possible. The sample is then kept at 4°C until tested within 3–4 h or frozen. When thawed the specimen should be tested immediately.

Method

Breakdown products are measured by crossed (two dimensional) immunoelectrophoresis. In the second dimension β globulins are electrophoresed into agarose containing anti-C3 (β1C/β1A). *See* Crossed Immunoelectrophoresis in Chapter 2 for technical details.

Comment

Normal serum gives one peak in the β1C position due to native C3. Any other peaks suggest the presence of breakdown products. A peak on the anodal side of C3 in the β1A position indicates C3c. The height of the peaks given by breakdown products is a measure of the quantity present.

If antiserum with activity against 'D' antigen is available, it may be used to detect C3d (α2D). The 'D' antigen is present on native C3, C3b and C3d. In crossed immunoelectrophoresis C3d may be detected as a peak on the anodal side of C3c.

Measurement of C3NeF

Method

C3 inactivators such as C3NeF may be detected by adding 1 vol of patient's serum to 1 vol of fresh normal serum which acts as a source of native C3 and incubating for 60 min at 37°C. The degree of C3 conversion can be evaluated by crossed immunoelectrophoresis using anti-C3 (β1C/β1A) antiserum.

Controls
(i) 1 vol patient's serum + 1 vol buffer; (ii) 1 vol normal serum + 1 vol buffer.

Comment
Differences between the test and controls indicate the quantity of C3NeF present. Measure the height of the peaks given by breakdown products in the patient's serum, in normal serum and in normal serum mixed with patient's serum. If the sum of the height of the peaks given by breakdown products in the mixture of patient's serum and normal serum exceeds that given by the sum of the peaks in individual samples from the patient and normal control, C3NeF is considered to be present.

Standardization of complement assays
As with any clinical laboratory test it is important that a study of normal individuals be undertaken so that the normal range can be defined for the population served by the laboratory as the first step towards producing a rational interpretation of patients' results.

INTERPRETATION OF COMPLEMENT PROFILE

Estimations of individual complement components only indicate the serum level at a single point in time and the result is the outcome of complement production, utilization, sequestration in tissues and catabolism. High levels could indicate increased production or a reduction in utilization or catabolism. Conversely low complement levels may reflect reduced production, deposition in tissues, or increased utilization. Levels within the normal range may occur when production is matched by utilization whether the overall turnover is depressed, normal or increased. These considerations are not always appreciated and it is tempting to take levels of any serum factor at face value without considering the dynamic situation. Complement turnover studies may elucidate these questions but are too complex for routine use.

To some extent difficulties of interpretation are overcome by studying profiles of selected components and repeating them later during the course of the illness to determine a pattern. In some cases assay of complement breakdown products may be helpful.

The serum components of complement most commonly assayed in patients with renal disorders are probably C1q, C4, C3, C3PA and properdin. C3 is depressed in several forms of glomerulonephritis and the levels of C1q and C4 give some indication of whether or not the classical complement pathway has been involved. It is worth repeating that a low C3 level in serum may not be due to increased utilization but may also be due to reduced production. A low C3 with low C1q and C4 indicates activation of the classical complement pathway and implies triggering by antigen-antibody complexes. A low C3 associated with normal C1q and C4 levels suggest activation of the alternative pathway. Depressed serum Factor B (C3PA) and properdin levels indicate alternative pathway activation.

Inherited deficiencies of particular complement components also occur and should not be overlooked. Family studies will be required to confirm the defect. Deficiencies of C1, C4 and C2 are often associated with diseases resembling systemic lupus erythematosus (Agnello, 1978).

SERUM COMPLEMENT PATTERNS IN PARTICULAR RENAL DISORDERS

Although the complement profile is not static during the course of an illness, characteristic patterns are frequently seen in specific renal diseases (Table 3.3).

Table 3.3 Serum complement profiles in renal diseases

Disorder	C1q	C4	C3	C3PA	Properdin
Minimal change disease	N	N	N	N	N
Acute proliferative glomerulonephritis	N or ↓	N or ↓	↓	N or ↓	↓
Mesangioproliferative glomerulonephritis	N	N	N	N	N
Mesangiocapillary glomerulonephritis					
Type I (Subendothelial deposits)	↓	↓	↓	↓	↓
Type II (Intramembranous deposits)	N	N	↓	N	N
Membranous glomerulonephritis	N	N	N	N	N
Systemic lupus erythematosus	↓	↓	↓	N or ↓	N or ↓
Goodpasture's syndrome	N	N	N	N	N
Focal glomerulosclerosis	N	N	↓	N	N
IgA nephropathy	N	N	N	N	N
Henoch-Schönlein syndrome	N	N	N	N	N
Renal graft rejection	↓	↓	↓	N	N
Haemolytic uraemic syndrome	N	N	N or ↓	N	N

In minimal change disease, complement levels are usually normal although low C1q levels have been found as an isolated finding in children with idiopathic nephrotic syndrome.

In acute proliferative glomerulonephritis, there is sometimes an acute phase response tending to elevate C3. Total haemolytic complement decreases as does C3 and C4. Concurrently the alternative pathway may be activated and C4 levels may become normal while a low C3 persists. In uncomplicated cases C3 levels return to normal in about 8–12 weeks. Renal biopsy reveals deposition of IgG and IgM in the glomerular basement membrane and C1q and C3 deposition. Factor B and properdin may also be detected.

In mesangioproliferative glomerulonephritis, there is no significant change in serum complement. Immunoglobulins, in particular IgM, and C3 may be deposited in the glomerulus.

In mesangiocapillary glomerulonephritis with subendothelial deposits (Type I), the serum levels of C3, C1q and C4 may all be reduced indicating activation of the conventional pathway. Factor B and properdin may be reduced and with the detection of C3NeF confirm alternative pathway activation. Affected kidneys show deposition of immune complexes within capillary loops associated with C3 deposition. Serum C3 is not usually as persistently low as it is in dense deposit disease and tends to become normal during the course of the disease (Habib & Levy, 1976). In mesangiocapillary glomerulonephritis with dense intramembranous deposits (Type II or dense deposit disease), a low C3 is usually accompanied by normal C1q and C4 levels. C3NeF is usually present. Glomeruli may show only complement deposition.

In membranous glomerulonephritis, complement profiles are usually within the normal range. Kidney biopsies show deposition of immune complexes in capillary walls staining for IgG, IgM and IgA together with C1q, C4 and C3.

In systemic lupus erythematosus, serum haemolytic complement activity, C3 and C4 are depressed and there is prominent deposition of immunoglobulins and C3 together with C1q and C4 in glomeruli, both in the mesangium and in capillary loops. Serum C3PA and properdin are decreased in some patients.

In Goodpasture's syndrome, significant changes are not usually seen in serum complement. Antibody mainly of the IgG type is deposited along the basement membrane of capillaries in the glomeruli and the alveolar walls of the lung, and is often accompanied by C3.

In focal glomerulosclerosis, serum C3 is sometimes depressed but other complement components are usually within the normal range. IgM and C3 are frequently deposited in the glomerulus.

In IgA nephropathy, serum C3 is not usually depressed and C1q and C4 are normal. IgA together with C3 and frequently IgG are deposited in the mesangium.

In Henoch-Schönlein syndrome, serum complement levels are usually within the normal range.

In renal graft rejection, C3 and C4 are frequently depressed along with C1q.

In the haemolytic uraemic syndrome, C3 depression is sometimes found.

Comment

Although the pathways of complement activation are complex and the picture is incomplete, simple techniques such as radial immunodiffusion and more recently the application of the Laurell rocket method permit the estimation of individual complement components with reasonable accuracy by all routine laboratories. The diagnostic value of complement estimation is seen particularly in acute glomerulonephritis, mesangiocapillary glomerulonephritis, systemic lupus erythematosus and renal graft rejection.

REFERENCES

Angello V 1978 Complement deficiency states. Medicine 57: 1–23
Davis A E, Arnaout M A, Alper C A, Rosen F S 1977 Transfer of C3 nephritic factor from mother to fetus. Is C3 nephritic factor IgG? New England Journal of Medicine 297: 144–145
Fothergill J E, Anderson W H K 1978 A molecular approach to the complement system. Current Topics in Cellular Regulation 13: 259–311
Habib R, Levy M 1976 Clinicopathologic correlations in 128 cases of membranoproliferative glomerulonephritis (MPGN). In: Proceedings of 6th International Congress of Nephrology Florence 1975: p 462–467 Karger, Basel

Lachmann P J, Hobart M J 1978 Complement technology. In: Handbook of Experimental Immunology ed Weir D M 3rd edn. vol. 1: Immunochemistry ch 5A Blackwell, Oxford

Laurell C-B 1972 Electroimmuno assay. Scandinavian Journal of Clinical Laboratory Investigation 29: suppl 124, 21–37

Mayer M M 1961 Complement and complement fixation. In Experimental Immunochemistry ed Kabat E A, Mayer M M ch 4 Thomas, Springfield

Müller-Eberhard H J 1975 Complement. Annual Review of Biochemistry 44: 697–724

Scott D M, Amos N, Sissons J G P, Lachmann P J, Peters D K 1978 The immunoglobulin nature of nephritic factor (NeF). Clinical and Experimental Immunology 32: 12–24

Spitzer R E, Vallota E H, Forristal J, Sudora E, Stitzel A, Davis N C, West C D 1969 Serum C′3 lytic system in patients with glomerulonephritis. Science 164: 436–437

Strong W M, Lea D J, Ward D J 1978 Measurement of total haemolytic complement activity in body fluids. Journal of Clinical Pathology 31: 527–530

UNCITED BIBLIOGRAPHY

Thompson R A 1977 Complement in perspective. In: Immunology in Medicine ed Holborow E J, Reeves W G ch 7 Academic Press, London

West C D 1976 Pathogenesis and approaches to therapy of membranoproliferative glomerulonephritis. Kidney International 9: 1–7

4

Immune Complexes

J. S. Hunt and A. R. McGiven

The kidney is affected more than any other organ by immune complexes which appear to be responsible for many forms of glomerulonephritis. This is partly explained by the fact that 20% of the cardiac output passes through the kidney and circulating complexes are trapped during glomerular filtration. This leads to the activation of mediators including complement and if persistent can result in extensive damage.

Immune complexes are formed in response to many infectious agents but in only a comparatively few instances do they lead to significant renal disease. The precise criteria which determine their pathogenicity are not well defined. It may depend on such factors as the nature of the antigen, the strength of the individual's immune response, the competence of the reticuloendothelial system and the ability of the kidney to clear immune complexes via the subendothelial-mesangial pathway. The avidity of the antibody, its immunoglobulin class and the net charge of the complex may also be of importance.

Antigen–antibody complexes may be formed whenever the reactive components are present and the size of the complex is determined by the relative concentration of each. It is important that the antigen and antibody have at least two binding sites for complexes to form aggregates. When present in equivalent proportions the complexes form particulate aggregates which will be removed by the reticuloendothelial system. When antigen is present in excess, small soluble immune complexes form. These are pathogenic and may lodge in the kidney.

DETECTION OF CIRCULATING IMMUNE COMPLEXES

Many methods have been developed to detect immune complexes in serum, and a brief review of the principle techniques is given below. Some methods depend on the physical and chemical characteristics of immune complexes while others depend on their biological properties. The following techniques do not require the antigen to be identified and do not provide information about the specific antigen and antibody involved in the reaction.

Physical techniques

Ultracentrifugation and gel filtration techniques based on the size of the immune complexes have been used in analytical work in specific diseases but are too time consuming for routine use. Reduced solubility in the cold is used to detect the presence of cryoglobulins which have been shown to contain antigen-antibody complexes and complement factors but may also be associated with other proteins.

Immune complexes may be precipitated by low concentrations of poly-ethyleneglycol. By itself this technique is rather nonspecific but is useful when associated with the detection of immunoglobulin and complement components by techniques such as liquid phase C1q binding or conglutinin binding.

Complement-dependent tests

The ability of immune complexes to activate the complement system is widely utilized and can be reflected by a decrease in total haemolytic complement activity and in individual complement components. Alternatively the ability of immune complexes to react with C1 through binding to its C1q component can be utilized.

C1q deviation

In the C1q deviation test, immune complexes compete with sensitized red cells for radiolabelled C1q. The radioactivity of the centrifuged red cell deposit is compared in the test and control samples and expressed as a percentage inhibition. This is a sensitive test but may be influenced by DNA and some bacterial products.

C1q precipitation

C1q if present in sufficient quantity will bind and precipitate immune complexes and aggregated γ globulin in agarose. This test is simple but is sensitive to DNA and polyanions and has been superseded.

C1q binding

In liquid phase C1q binding, the patient's serum is incubated with radiolabelled C1q. Free C1q and C1q bound in immune complexes are separated by differential precipitation by polyethylene glycol. The percentage of radioactive C1q precipitated is a measure of the complexes present.

In solid phase C1q binding, C1q is coated on to polystyrene tubes and incubated with the test serum. After washing, radioactive labelled anti-IgG is added and binds to the immunoglobulin of complexes which have bound to the C1q on the tube. This is the particular method which our own laboratory favours and details will be given below.

Some C1q binding methods require heat inactivation of the serum to inhibit C1q and this may lead to the formation of globulin aggregates. In the method outlined in detail in this chapter, C1q in test serum is inactivated by treatment with EDTA.

C1q can react with aggregates of globulin whether these are formed spontaneously or from repeated freezing and thawing. Other substances which may react with C1q are polyanions including endotoxin polysaccharide and single and double stranded DNA.

In spite of these shortcomings C1q binding assays remain among the most popular of tests for immune complexes and are capable of detecting complexes of both the IgG and IgM types.

Rheumatoid factor and related tests

Rheumatoid factor, 19S antiIgG will precipitate immune complexes in agarose. It is done best by monoclonal rheumatoid factor from patients with lymphoproliferative disorders rather than the polyclonal rheumatoid factor obtained from patients with rheumatoid arthritis.

Tests based on the inhibition by immune complexes of the binding of rheumatoid factor to aggregated immunoglobulin have also been developed.

These tests have the defect that rheumatoid factor may be present in the patient's serum and interfere with the test.

Binding to cell surface receptors

Platelet aggregation

Immune complexes bind to the surfaces of platelets leading to aggregate formation. Platelets prepared from fresh blood are added to serial dilutions of the test sera. The preparation is read after overnight incubation at 4°C. A small button is a negative result. A diffuse carpet is a positive result. The test suffers from individual variations in the reactions of platelets and three different preparations of platelets are used with aggregated human IgG as a positive control.

Raji test

The Raji lymphoblastoid cell line, derived from Burkitt's lymphoma, has surface receptors for C3 and has been used successfully to detect immune complexes. The complexes bind to the cell membrane via the complement receptor and are recognized by a radiolabelled anti-human globulin serum. Quantitation is obtained by referring to a standard curve prepared using various amounts of aggregated globulin. It is one of the most sensitive tests but suffers from the defect that the Raji cell culture line must be maintained and there is some variation in the background binding of cells used at different times (Woodroffe et al, 1977). Lymphocytotoxic antibodies commonly found in patients with systemic lupus erythematosus may interfere with the test.

Inhibition of complement-dependent lymphocyte rosettes

The binding of complement coated erythrocytes to lymphocyte complement receptors may be inhibited by the complement associated with immune complexes.

Inhibition of macrophage ingestion

This test is based on the inhibition by immune complexes of the uptake of radiolabelled immunoglobulin aggregates by guinea-pig peritoneal macrophages.

Which test?

The above wide-ranging selection of tests for circulating immune complexes based on physicochemical and biological characteristics is in itself an indication that no single test is entirely satisfactory for diagnostic purposes.

Many of the tests measure globulin aggregates regardless of whether antigen is present and in themselves are not specific for immune complexes. As aggregation may arise spontaneously, or from freezing and thawing of serum this is always a potential source of error. In some cases, rheumatoid factor may contribute to erroneous interpretation while in others native complement and polyanionic substances including DNA and endotoxin polysaccharide may be responsible.

As the tests depend on different characteristics of immune complexes it is not surprising that different tests will give different results on the same sample of serum. At present there is no single straightforward laboratory test which can be advocated for the routine detection of immune complexes. Laboratories investigating immune complexes have tended to develop at least one and often two tests from the C1q binding, monoclonal rheumatoid factor precipitation and Raji cell groups and have supplemented this with functional complement assays.

C1q tests depend on complement binding by the classical pathway and have the disadvantage of reacting with non-immune substances such as aggregated globulin.

Monoclonal rheumatoid factor precipitation occurs with the smaller soluble complexes which are not cleared by the reticuloendothelial system. Although it only reacts with IgG, this is no serious disadvantage.

The Raji test has the problem of maintaining the lymphoblastoid cell culture and lymphocytoxic antibodies affect the test.

All methods have the problem of standardization between different test runs.

Two tests are described in detail below. One is a functional assay of anti-complementary activity. The other is a solid phase C1q binding radioimmuno-assay.

IMMUNE COMPLEX DETECTION FROM ANTICOMPLEMENTARY ACTIVITY

The ability of immune complexes to bind complement is utilized in this test. A standard amount of guinea-pig complement is added to heat-inactivated test serum and, following fixation by immune complexes present, residual complement activity is estimated using a standard haemolytic system. The heating inactivates any complement which may have been already bound to complexes in the patient's serum. From the back titration of guinea-pig complement, the loss of haemolytic activity can be calculated.

Equipment
Measuring cylinder 250 ml—Centrifuge tubes 2 (to wash sheep erythrocytes)—Beaker 25 ml × 2 (for sheep erythrocytes and complement)—Conical flask 50 ml —Test tubes 12 × 75 mm—Pipettes 2 ml, 5 ml, 10 ml—Micropipette to deliver 0.10 and 0.20 ml (Oxford microdiluter)—Pasteur pipettes—Spectrophotometer —Glass microcuvettes 1 ml—Parafilm—Waterbath 56°C—Graph paper.

Reagents
Complement-fixing diluent tablets, veronal buffer pH 7.2 (Oxoid)—Distilled water—Guinea-pig complement—Sheep erythrocytes—Normal saline—Haemolysin—rabbit anti-sheep erythrocyte serum (Wellcome).

Method

Titration of haemolysin and complement. Determine the HD50 dilution of the batch of complement and the optimum sensitizing concentration of haemolysin by standard checkerboard titration. In practice a haemolysin dilution of 1 : 150 or 1 : 200 is usually satisfactory and the complement dilution can then be determined by a one row series of dilutions rather than the full checkerboard procedure.

Sensitization of sheep erythrocytes. Wash the sheep erythrocytes three times in saline and then add 1 ml of packed cells to 19 ml of reconstituted buffer and mix. Add 0.1 ml of haemolysin to 19.9 ml of complement-fixing buffer and mix. Add the 20 ml of washed sheep erythrocytes to the 20 ml of diluted haemolysin, mix gently and place in a waterbath at 37°C for 30 min. Mix after 15 and 30 min. The sensitized sheep cells can be kept at 4°C overnight if necessary until required.

Preparation of standard complement dilutions. Dilute the complement with complement-fixing buffer to give 6HD50 units/ml. Then prepare the following dilutions—

Tube	6HD50 units ml	Complement-fixing buffer ml	Total HD50 units
1	2.0	2.0	3.0
2	1.0	1.4	2.5
3	1.0	2.0	2.0
4	1.0	2.3	1.8
5	1.0	2.8	1.6
6	1.0	3.3	1.4
7	0.5	2.0	1.2
8	0.5	2.2	1.1
9	0.5	2.5	1.0
10	0.5	2.8	0.9
11	0.5	3.3	0.8
12	0.25	1.9	0.7
13	0.25	2.3	0.6
14	0.25	2.8	
15	0.0	1.0	0.0 (Blank)

Thereafter—

(*i*) Take 15 test tubes and transfer 0.1 ml of the above complement dilutions to the appropriate tube.

(*ii*) Add 0.1 ml of complement-fixing buffer to each and incubate at 4°C for 30 min.

(*iii*) Add 0.2 ml of sensitized sheep erythrocytes to each tube. Mix gently and incubate at 37°C for 15 min.

(*iv*) Dilute with 1 ml of complement-fixing buffer and mix.

(*v*) Centrifuge each tube for 5 min at 400 g.

(*vi*) Transfer the supernatants to clean test tubes and read the absorbance for each complement dilution on a spectrophotometer at 541 nm.

Test sera. Add 0.2 ml of each test serum to a glass test tube (A) and place in a waterbath at 56°C for 1 h to inactivate complement. Remove 0.1 ml of serum and place in another test tube (B). Add 0.1 ml of the 3HD50 complement dilution to tubes A (test). Add 0.1 ml of complement-fixing buffer to tubes B (blank). Incubate at 4°C for 30 min.—Add 0.2 ml of sensitized sheep red cells and continue as outlined above for the standard complement dilutions (*iii*).—When reading the absorbance, subtract each blank value from the test value to correct for colour in the serum.

Calculation of anticomplementary activity. Construct a reference curve by plotting the absorbance at 541 nm against the HD50 units of the control dilution of complement. The graph is sigmoid shaped and one HD50 unit of complement should lyse 50% of the indicator cells. Read the HD50 values corresponding to the absorbance given by the test sera. This reading corresponds to the complement activity remaining after utilization by immune complexes or other mechanisms. As 3 HD50 units of complement were added, the observed value should be subtracted from 3 to give the units of complement which have been consumed.

Interpretation. The range of complement consumption in normal sera should be established for each laboratory by studying a group of healthy individuals. A result higher than the normal range is consistent with the presence of immune complexes.

Comment

This test suffers from a defect common to many tests in that aggregated immunoglobulin may fix complement. Sera with high IgG levels may give raised levels of complement consumption.

Anticomplementary tests have proved to be a useful practical aid in the detection and monitoring of antigen-antibody complexes and can be used to supplement other assays. They may be carried out by laboratories not equipped for more complex tests.

IMMUNE COMPLEX DETECTION BY C1q BINDING RADIOIMMUNOASSAY

This test depends on the binding of immune complexes in serum added to C1q-coated polystyrene test tubes. After washing out unbound proteins, ^{125}I labelled anti-human IgG is added to the tube and adheres to the IgG component of the immune complex which has bound by its Fc portion to adherent C1q. Excess radioactive anti-IgG is washed out and the remaining radioactivity measured in a gamma counter is an indirect measure of the immune complexes present.

The technique described below is based on that described by Hay et al (1976) and further modified by those workers. It detects only IgG immune complexes.

Preparation of C1q

The preparation of C1q is based on the method of Yonemasu & Stroud (1971). All solutions are prepared using deionized water of resistivity < 18 megohm/cm.

Equipment

Analytical balance—Hot plate magnetic stirrer—Conductivity meter—pH meter—Refrigerated centrifuge with swing out rotors for both large (4 × 250 ml) and small (5 × 50 ml) tubes, *e.g.* Sorvall RC 2B with HB 4 and HB 4 rotors—Immunoelectrophoresis equipment including levelling table, trough and well cutter, tank, cooling plate, power supply, humidity chamber, soaking and staining trays—Spectrophotometer and quartz cuvettes—Deep freeze −70°C —Deionized water apparatus—Beakers 250 ml, 1 litre, 5 litre—Centrifuge bottles (250 ml) and tubes (50 ml) polycarbonate or polypropylene—Measuring pipettes 2 ml, 5 ml, 10 ml—Glass test tubes 6 × 25 mm, siliconized—Dialysis tubing—Waterbath at 63°C—Chromatography column 1.5 × 90 cm—Fraction collection apparatus.

Reagents

(*i*) *0.026M EGTA, pH 7.5, conductivity 3.48 mMho/cm.* 19.8 g EGTA is heated with approximately 200 ml of deionized water to about 60°C. Add 5M NaOH to pH 7.5 and then add deionized water until the correct conductivity is reached. This makes approximately 2 l of buffer.

(*ii*) *0.75M NaCl in 0.02M acetate buffer containing 0.01M EDTA, pH 5.0,* conductivity 71 mMho/cm.—(*a*) Dissolve 10.958 g NaCl, 0.93 g EDTA (disodium), 0.41 g sodium acetate in deionized water and make up to 250 ml. (*b*) Dissolve 10.958 g NaCl, 0.93 g EDTA (disodium), 0.285 ml glacial acetic acid in deionized water and make up to 250 ml. Add *b* to *a* to pH 5.0, then adjust conductivity.

(*iii*) *0.06M EDTA, pH 5.0, conductivity 7.25 mMho/cm.* Dissolve 89.3 g EDTA (disodium salt) in 3 litres of deionized water and adjust pH with 5M NaOH. Add deionized water to required conductivity. This makes 4 litres of buffer.

(*iv*) *0.75M NaCl in 0.005M phosphate buffer containing 0.01M EDTA, pH 7.5,* conductivity 71 mMho/cm. Dissolve 10.958 g NaCl, 0.93 g EDTA (disodium), 0.22 g Na$_2$HPO$_4$.2H$_2$O in deionized water and adjust pH with 5M NaOH. Make up to 250 ml and adjust conductivity.

(*v*) *0.035M EDTA, pH 7.5, conductivity 7.5 mMho/cm.* Dissolve 52.1 g EDTA (disodium salt) in 3 litres of deionized water and adjust pH with 5M NaOH. Add deionized water to required conductivity. This makes 4 litres of buffer.

(*vi*) *0.75M NaCl in 0.02M acetate buffer containing 0.01M EDTA, pH 7.5,* conductivity 71 mMho/cm. Elevate pH of buffer (*ii*) using 5M NaOH then adjust conductivity.

(*vii*) *0.1M phosphate buffer, pH 7.0,* conductivity 15 mMho/cm. (*a*) Dissolve 13.61 g KH$_2$PO$_4$ in deionized water and make up to 1 litre. (*b*) Dissolve 17.79 g Na$_2$HPO$_4$ in deionized water and make up to 1 litre. Add approximately 400 ml of *a* to approximately 600 ml *b* to pH 7.0 then adjust conductivity.

Method

Collect 300 ml of normal human blood. Allow to clot for 60 min at room temperature and let the clot retract for 2 h at 4°C. Separate the serum by centrifugation at 4°C and 3000 *g* for 10 min and then recentrifuge at 4°C and 20 000 *g* for 90 min to remove free lipid. Aspirate the serum from below the lipid layer.

Dialyse 130 ml of the serum against 1 litre of 0.026M EGTA, pH 7.5, conductivity 3.48 mMho/cm at 4°C for 4 h. Renew the buffer and continue dialysis for a further 11 h.

Centrifuge at 4°C and 16 250 *g* for 10 min and wash the precipitate once with approximately 3 ml of fresh 0.026M EGTA buffer as above. Dissolve the precipitate in 32 ml of 0.75M NaCl in 0.02M acetate buffer containing 0.01M EDTA, pH 5.0, conductivity 71 mMho/cm. Centrifuge at 4°C and 16 250 *g* for 10 min and discard insoluble aggregates.

Dialyse the clear solution against 4 litres of 0.06M EDTA, pH 5.0, conductivity 7.25 mMho/cm at 4°C for 4 h. Separate the precipitate by centrifugation at 3000 *g* for 10 min, wash once with fresh 0.06M EDTA buffer and then dissolve the precipitate in 32 ml of 0.75M NaCl in 0.005 M phosphate buffer solution containing 0.01M EDTA, pH 7.5, conductivity 71 mMho/cm. Eliminate insoluble aggregates by centrifugation.

Dialyse the solution against 4 litres of 0.035M EDTA, pH 7.5, conductivity 7.5 mMho/cm at 4°C for 5 h. Separate the precipitate, wash once with fresh 0.035M EDTA buffer, then dissolve in a minimum (approximately 4 ml) vol. of 0.75M NaCl in 0.02M acetate buffer containing 0.01M EDTA, pH 7.5 conductivity 71 mMho/cm. Eliminate insoluble aggregates by centrifugation.

Dialyse the solution against 1 litre of 0.1M phosphate buffer, pH 7.0 conductivity 15 mMho/cm at 4°C for 4 h.

Establish the presence of C1q by Ouchterlony immunodiffusion and purity by immunoelectrophoresis against anti-human serum. Estimate the protein concentration by Lowry's method. *See* Chapter 2 for details of these methods. Aliquot and store at −70°C. Activity may diminish after two months in storage.

Note 1. Use polycarbonate centrifuge tubes and store C1q in siliconized glass as it adheres to other surfaces.

2. Times for dialysis are times to completion and may be left longer for convenience.

Preparation of ¹²⁵I affinity purified anti-human IgG

The purity and specificity of the anti-human globulin which is to be iodinated is an important consideration in this test. Some commercial preparations although containing antibodies of high specificity also contain buffering filler proteins which are not required for iodination. These unwanted proteins are removed by affinity chromatography.

It is recommended that the iodinated anti-IgG serum be directed only against the Fc portion of human IgG. However, useful results can be obtained using antisera directed against whole IgG.

Preparation of IgG

Equipment
Fraction collection apparatus—UV monitor—Peristaltic pump—Chromatography column 2.6 × 40 cm—pH meter—Freeze dryer—Magnetic stirrer—Beakers 1 litre, 5 litre—Deep freeze −20°C—Deionized water apparatus—Dialysis tubing 15 mm, 20 mm diameter.

Reagents
QAE Sephadex A50—NaOH 5M—0.1M Tris-HCl buffer pH 6.6, prepared by dissolving 12.1 g Tris (hydroxymethyl) methylamine in 950 ml of deionized water, adjusting pH to 6.6 with concentrated HCl, and making up to 1 litre with deionized water.

Method
IgG sufficient for linking to Sepharose and for forming aggregates for standardization can be separated from 15–20 ml of human serum by ion exchange chromatography on a 2.6 × 40 cm column of QAE Sephadex A50.

Soak 8 g of QAE Sephadex A50 (Pharmacia) in 750 ml of 0.1M Tris-HCl buffer pH 6.6. Adjust the pH to 6.6 with a few drops of 5M NaOH. Allow the gel to swell for 2–3 h then remove the supernatant and wash with a further 750 ml of buffer. Dialyse the serum sample for 2–3 h against buffer before loading on the column of this gel. Load the sample on the column and elute with 0.1M Tris-HCl buffer pH 6.6 at 18–20 ml/h. Pool tubes from the first peak and dialyse extensively against deionized water to remove buffer before freeze drying. Store desiccated at −20°C.

Isolation of specific anti-human IgG

Equipment
Quickfit scintered glass funnel 250 ml—Quickfit side arm Erlenmeyer flask 500 ml—Vacuum source—Cold laboratory 4°C—Fraction collection apparatus—UV monitor—Peristaltic pump—Syringe 5 ml with attached silicon rubber tubing—Pressure concentrating cell—Immunoelectrophoresis equipment—Magnetic stirrer—Glass test tubes 6 × 25 mm, siliconized—Conductivity meter—pH meter—Deionized water apparatus.

Reagents
CNBr-activated Sepharose 4B and coupling reagents—Human IgG—Phosphate-buffered saline 0.1M pH 7.3 Dulbecco A (PBS)—Rabbit anti-human IgG (Dakopatts, Denmark)—Lowry reagents for protein determination—Sodium azide—Dialysis tubing—Phosphate buffer 0.1M, pH 7.0 conductivity 15 mMho/cm—Glycine buffer 0.2M glycine, 0.5M NaCl pH 2.8, prepared by dissolving 15 g glycine and 29.25 g NaCl in 950 ml distilled water, adjusting pH to 2.8 with concentrated HCl, and making up to 1 litre with distilled water.

Method
Human IgG is coupled by standard methods to CNBr-activated Sepharose 4B

(Pharmacia) and packed into a 5 ml syringe, then kept at 4°C with 0.02% sodium azide as preservative.

Connect column to a fraction collector in the cold room and equilibrate with phosphate-buffered saline (PBS).

Dialyse 5 ml rabbit anti-human IgG against 1 litre of PBS at 4°C for 4h. The amount of anti-IgG added to the column depends upon the quantity required and column volume; 5 ml should last at least six months.

Load the sample on to the prepared Sepharose column and allow binding to occur for 1 h.

Elute unbound protein with PBS until the absorbance indicates this is complete.

Elute the specific anti-human IgG with 0.2M glycine buffer containing 0.5M NaCl, pH 2.8. Neutralize the solution of eluted antibody by adding about two drops of 1M NaOH to each of the tubes from this second peak. Pool these tubes, adjust pH to 7.0–7.5 and then concentrate to about 3 mg/ml.

Determine the antibody activity by Ouchterlony immunodiffusion and protein concentration by Lowry's method. (It should be possible to combine this preparation with a preparation of C1q and do a Lowry protein estimation simultaneously).

Dialyse against 0.1M phosphate buffer, pH 7.0, conductivity 15 mMho/cm at 4°C for 4h. The protein is then ready to be labelled and/or stored at −70°C in siliconized glass tubes.

Iodination of antihuman IgG

Equipment
Fume cupboard designed for use with radioisotopes—Gamma counter—Fraction collection apparatus—Chromatography column 0.9×15 cm—Micropipettes: 20 μl; 50 μl—Balance—pH meter—Glass test tubes 6×25 mm, siliconized—Deep freeze −70°C—Spectrophotometer and quartz microcuvettes 1 ml capacity—Glass test tubes 12×15 mm—Pasteur pipettes—Latex gloves

Reagents
   (i) *^{125}I NaI 100 mCi/ml in NaOH, pH 7–11* (Amersham IMS 30).
  (ii) *Sephadex G50.*
 (iii) *Phosphate-buffered saline pH 7.3 Dulbecco A (PBS).*
 (iv) *Phosphate buffer 0.5M pH 7.4* (a) Dissolve 6.80 g KH_2PO_4 in 100 ml distilled water. (b) Dissolve 8.89 g Na_2HPO_4 in 100 ml distilled water. Add approximately 20 ml of solution *a* to 80 ml of solution *b* to pH 7.4.
   (v) *Chloramine T.* Dissolve 20 mg in 10 ml of 0.5M phosphate buffer pH 7.4.
  (vi) *Sodium metabisulphite.* Dissolve 20 mg in 10 ml of 0.5M phosphate buffer pH 7.4.
 (vii) *Potassium iodide.* Dissolve 10 mg in 10 ml of 0.5M phosphate buffer pH 7.4.
(viii) *Affinity purified anti-IgG.*

Method
The antibody is labelled with ^{125}I by the chloramine T method (Hunter, 1978). Iodination is performed in a 12×75 mm round bottomed glass tube on ice.

Add 20 μl of 0.5M phosphate buffer pH 7.4. Add 0.5 mCi [125]I (5 μl of NaI 100 mCi/ml in NaOH solution pH 7–11, Amersham IMS 30) and mix.

Add 200 μg of specific antibody (already in 100–200 μl of 0.1M phosphate buffer pH 7.0) and mix. Allow to cool on crushed ice.

Add 100 μg of Chloramine T (50 μl of 2 mg/ml solution in 0.5M phosphate buffer). Mix and leave 60 s on ice.

Add 100 μg of sodium metabisulphite (50 μl of 2 mg/ml solution in 0.5M phosphate buffer). Mix and leave 2 min on ice.

Add 50 μg potassium iodide (50 μl of 1 mg/ml solution in 0.5M phosphate buffer). Mix and leave on ice.

Free iodine is separated from protein-bound iodine on a Sephadex G50 column. Load the sample on to the column and elute with PBS (Dulbecco) at 4°C, collecting 0.5 ml fractions.

10 μl aliquots are counted on a gamma counter, tubes from the first peak pooled and then the protein absorbance measured at 280 nm. Protein concentration is obtained by reference to a standard curve prepared for rabbit IgG and specific activity calculated.

The labelled antibody is then aliquoted into amounts suitable for a single test run and stored at $-70°C$ in siliconized glass tubes.

C1q binding assay

Equipment
Refrigerator 4°C—Gamma counter—Polystyrene tubes 12×75 mm—Micropipettes: 50 μl; 100 μl—Graduated pipettes 1 ml—Glass tubes 12×75 mm—Water bath 37°C.

Reagents
Phosphate-buffered saline pH 7.3 Dulbecco A (PBS)—[125]I anti-human IgG—C1q 10 μg/ml in PBS—0.1% gelatine in PBS—0.05% Tween 20 in PBS—EDTA 0.2M pH 7.5, prepared by dissolving 7.44 g EDTA disodium salt in 90 ml of deionized water, adjusting pH to 7.5 with 5M NaOH, and making up to 100 ml with deionized water.

Method
Preparation of C1q coated polystyrene tubes. (*i*) Bind C1q to polystyrene tubes by adding 10 μg in 1 ml of PBS to each tube and incubate at 4°C for 3 d. (*ii*) Wash tubes 3 times with cold PBS then fill with 0.1% gelatine in PBS and incubate at room temperature for 2 h. (*iii*) Wash tubes $\times 3$ with cold PBS.— The tubes are now ready to be used in the assay and may be stored at 4°C for up to two weeks. Serum samples to be assayed are stored at $-20°C$ until required.

Assay procedure. (*i*) Mix 50 μl test serum with 100 μl 0.2M EDTA, pH 7.5 in a glass tube and incubate at 37°C for 30 min. Transfer mixture to an ice bath. (*ii*) Place duplicate 50 μl EDTA-treated samples in the C1q-coated tubes together with 950 μl of PBS containing 0.05% Tween-20 (PBS-Tween). Incubate tubes at 37°C for 1 h and at 4°C for 30 min. (*iii*) Wash unbound proteins from the tubes by filling and emptying three times with cold PBS. (*iv*) Add 1 μg of ^{125}I-labelled rabbit anti-human IgG in 1 ml PBS-Tween to tubes and incubate at 37°C for 1 h and at 4°C for 30 min. (*v*) Remove unbound labelled antibody by washing $\times 3$ with cold PBS. (*vi*) Count tubes in a gamma ray spectrometer.

Standards. Prepare two standards containing 1 μg ^{125}I-labelled rabbit anti-human IgG in 1 ml PBS-Tween in an uncoated polystyrene tube and count. The results of the assay are expressed in terms of these counts.

Background controls. Prepare two background controls in the same manner as test serum samples but add 1 ml PBS-Tween in place of serum plus 950 μl PBS-Tween.

Controls. In each run of assay include a positive and two normal controls in duplicate.

Calculation of results. The number of counts remaining in each tube is expressed as nanograms of anti-IgG. This is calculated from the standards containing 1 μg of anti-IgG. The number of nanograms of anti-IgG bound by the tubes containing the test samples is then calculated by subtracting the value for the background control from test samples values.

Standardization of assay

Aggregated human IgG may be used to provide a standardized C1q binding reagent for comparison between different batches of C1q. However, aggregated IgG appears to be rather unstable on storage and should be kept at -70°C for not longer than four weeks. Fresh preparations of aggregated IgG have shown consistent binding up to a concentration of 25 μg/ml aggregated IgG with batches of C1q.

Preparation of aggregated IgG

Equipment

Spectrophotometer and quartz cuvettes—Refrigerated centrifuge and tubes, polycarbonate 30×100 mm—Water bath at 63°C—Chromatography column 1.5×90 cm—Fraction collection apparatus—Ultracentrifuge, swing out rotor and tubes, polyallomer 13×50 mm—Deep freeze -70°C—Glass test tubes 6×25 mm, siliconized.

Reagents

NaOH 0.1M—Phosphate-buffered saline pH 7.3 Dulbecco A (PBS)—Ultrogel AcA 34—Bovine serum albumin (lyophilized)—Human IgG.

Method

Dissolve 50 mg human IgG in 1 ml PBS. This will require the pH of the solution to be raised to 8.0-9.0 using 0.1M NaOH. Centrifuge at 2500g for 10 min to remove insoluble material.

Measure absorbance at 280 nm and calculate the concentration from a standard curve for human IgG. Dilute the solution to approximately 25 mg/ml in PBS. Incubate at 63°C for 20 min. Cool immediately to 0°C.

Centrifuge at 4°C and 25 000 g for 10 min. Remove supernatant.

Remove non-aggregated IgG by running the solution on a column of Ultrogel AcA 34 and eluting with PBS.

Pool tubes containing aggregated IgG, then centrifuge at 4°C and 150 000 g for 1 h to obtain pellet of aggregate. (Beckman ultracentrifuge: rotor SW 50.1 at 36 000 RPM).

Dissolve the pellet in 1 ml PBS and measure the absorbance at 280 nm for protein concentration. Add bovine serum albumin to 2% (w/v) and adjust the pH to 8.0 with 0.1 M NaOH.

Store at -70°C in siliconized glass for up to four weeks. Centrifuge at 1000 g for 10 min prior to use to eliminate large aggregates.

Standard curve for assay should be made using aggregated human IgG for each new batch of C1q and rabbit anti-human IgG used in the assay. This is prepared by adding 1 μg, 5 μg, 10 μg, 25 μg and 50 μg aggregated IgG in duplicate to C1q coated tubes in 1 ml PBS-Tween, in place of the test serum sample. A curve is drawn plotting μg of aggregated IgG added against ng of rabbit anti-human IgG bound.

Interpretation

Although the preparation of reagents for the C1q binding assay reads as a lengthy and complicated process, in practice it is within the ability of most laboratories which undertake radioimmunoassays and have facilities for standard protein chemistry techniques.

Once C1q and affinity purified ^{125}I anti-human IgG have been prepared the test procedure is simple and batches of sera can be tested within a few hours. Fresh batches of C1q should be prepared at intervals of about two months. Aliquots of anti-human IgG sera require labelling with ^{125}I at intervals of about one month.

The difficulties of having absolute standardization between one test run and another, particularly those where different reagents have been used are not always overcome in practice. It is probably best to regard the test as semi-quantitative and to relate the results to a range of normal sera run in the same batch as the test sera. Some laboratories may find that a four point scale of normal, doubtful, positive and strongly positive is the most satisfactory method of reporting the results both for the purposes of diagnosis and also for monitoring clinical progress.

Micromethod solid phase C1q binding assay

Our laboratory has converted the above tube technique to a micromethod. Whereas the quantity of C1q from 300 ml blood permits about 80 samples to be assayed by the tube technique, with a tenfold reduction in the volumes used, nearly seven times as many assays, performed in triplicate, can be carried out by the micromethod. There is no loss of sensitivity and binding of C1q appears to be enhanced.

For the micromethod we prefer to use a more heavily ^{125}I-labelled rabbit anti-human-globulin (1.25 μCi/μg). *See* Iodination of Anti-human IgG. In the first step of the procedure add 12 μl NaI 100 mCi/ml (and not 5 μl as specified for use with the tube method). This is the only modification in the preparation of reagents. Plastic plates from different manufacturers vary in their binding of C1q and also in the ease with which individual wells can be separated for counting. Microtitre system plates with round bottom wells (Cooke M220–24 AR, Germany) are satisfactory.

Method

Preparation of plates. Add 100 μl of C1q (10 μg/ml in PBS) to each well in the microtitre plate. Cover and keep at 4°C for three days. Wash each well $\times 3$ with 200 μl cold PBS. Add 200 μl 0.1 % gelatine-PBS solution, cover and leave at room temperature for 2 h. Wash wells $\times 3$ with 200 μl cold PBS. Drain and allow to dry at room temperature. Cover and store at 4°C until required.

Assay procedure.
(*i*) Add 50 μl of test sera to 100 μl of 0.2M EDTA pH 7.5 in glass tubes and incubate at 37°C for 30 min. Transfer tubes to an ice bath.
(*ii*) From each test tube take triplicate 5 μl samples and place in C1q coated wells.
(*iii*) Add 100 μl PBS containing 0.05 % Tween-20 to each well.
(*iv*) Cover and incubate plates at 37°C for 1 h and at 4°C for 30 min.
(*v*) Remove unbound proteins by washing wells $\times 3$ with 200 μl cold PBS.
(*vi*) Add 0.1 μg ^{125}I-labelled rabbit antihuman IgG in 100 μl PBS-Tween 20 and incubate at 37°C for 1 h and at 4°C for 30 min.
(*vii*) Remove unbound labelled antibody by washing $\times 3$ with 200 μl of cold PBS. Drain and allow to dry.
(*viii*) In preparation for counting remove all wells from the plate by cutting horizontally above the 100 μl level with a hot wire. Then snip off each well with scissors and place in a separate glass test tube for counting.

Controls are similar to those for the tube method. In preparing the standard curve for binding by aggregated globulin, 100 μl samples are used.

IMMUNE COMPLEX RENAL DISEASE

The incidence of immune complexes compiled from a review of a variety of tests in the literature is given in Table 4.1. Immune complexes have been found in the sera of patients with minimal change disease, acute proliferative glomerulonephritis, focal glomerulonephritis and lupus nephritis. In lupus nephritis there seems to be a good relationship between activity of the disease and the detection of immune complexes in the serum. Negative results have often been obtained in Goodpasture's syndrome and in some reports, IgA nephropathy and membranous nephritis have given negative results with C1q and Raji tests.

At first sight it is rather anomalous that a disease such as membraneous nephritis which from immunofluorescence and electron microscopic appearance is clearly associated with the deposition of immune complexes in the kidney is

Table 4.1. Incidence of immune complexes in serum

Renal disorder	% positive
Acute poststreptococcal glomerulonephritis	80–90
Mesangiocapillary glomerulonephritis	30–50
Mesangioproliferative glomerulonephritis	20
Membranous glomerulonephritis	30
Minimal change disease	25–50
Focal glomerulosclerosis	50
Systemic lupus erythematosus	50–80
Renal transplant	60–70
Polyarteritis nodosa	30–70
Goodpasture's syndrome	25
Henoch-Schönlein syndrome	30
IgA nephropathy	30

frequently not shown to have circulating immune complexes. Conversely the demonstration of circulating immune complexes in a significant proportion of patients with minimal change disease contrasts with the failure to localize deposits in the kidney by immunofluorescence or electron microscopy.

The detection of immune complexes depends on the timing of the investigation. Not only may variable results be due to different techniques but also to the failure to test the patient when complexes are present in the circulation. Findings from immune complex assays should be correlated with the results of other investigations such as the serum complement profile and tests of renal function.

Nature of the antigen
Although immune complexes have been implicated in many forms of renal disease particularly glomerulonephritis, in the majority of patients the antigen is not usually known. However in a number of isolated cases certain antigens have been recognized. Bacterial antigens have been identified in acute diffuse proliferative glomerulonephritis, shunt nephritis and focal embolic nephritis complicating bacterial endocarditis. Hepatitis B, P. malariae and S. mansoni have also been implicated. A list of micro-organisms involved in immune complex disorders is given at the beginning of the next chapter. DNA antigens have been identified in lupus nephritis, and in a few cases of immune complex glomerulonephritis thyroid antigens have been identified.

In most cases of membranous and mesangiocapillary nephritis, the antigen remains unknown. Occasionally some patients have suffered from malignant tumours and tumour antigens have been detected in the kidney.

REFERENCES

Hay F C, Nineham L J, Roitt I M 1976 Routine assay for the detection of immune complexes of known immunoglobulin class using solid phase C1q. Clinical and Experimental Immunology 24: 396–400

Hunter W M 1978 Radioimmunoassay. In: Handbook of Experimental Immunology ed Weir D M 3rd edn. vol 1: Immunochemistry ch 14 Blackwell, Oxford

Lowry O H, Rosebrough N J, Farr A L, Randall R J 1951 Protein measurement with the Folin phenol reagent. Journal of Biological Chemistry 193: 265–275

Woodroffe A J, Border W A, Theofilopoulos A N, Götze O, Glassock R J, Dixon F J, Wilson
C B 1977 Detection of circulating immune complexes in patients with glomerulonephritis.
Kidney International 12: 268–278
Yonemasu K, Stroud R M 1971 C1q: Rapid purification method for preparation of monospecific
antisera and for biochemical studies. Journal of Immunology 106: 304–313

UNCITED BIBLIOGRAPHY

McCluskey R T, Hall C L, Colvin R B 1978 Immune complex mediated diseases. Human
Pathology, 9: 71–84
Ooi Y M, Vallota E H, West C D 1977 Serum immune complexes in membranoproliferative and
other glomerulonephritides. Kidney International 11: 275–283
Woodroffe A J, Foldes M, McKenzie P E, Thompson A J, Seymour A E, Clarkson A R 1979
Serum immune complexes and disease. Australian and New Zealand Journal of Medicine 9:
129–135
Zubler R H, Lambert P H 1977 Immune complexes in clinical investigation. In: Recent Advances
in Clinical Immunology ed Thompson R A ch 6 Churchill Livingstone, Edinburgh

5
Antibodies and Autoantibodies
A. R. McGiven

A variety of antibodies occur in patients with renal disease. Some bacterial antibodies indicate the probable nature of a particular disease process affecting the kidney while others indicate the co-existence of bacterial infections which are likely to occur in patients with reduced resistance to infection either because of the nature of their renal disease or as a result of immunosuppressive therapy.

The organisms implicated in renal disease include—

Immune complex disorders
Bacteria. Streptococci; Staphylococci; Pneumococci; C. bovis; S. typhi; M. leprae; T. pallidum; Enterococci.
   Parasites. P. malariae; P. falciparum; S. mansoni; T. gondii.
   Viruses. Hepatitis B; Measles; Epstein Barr; Oncorna virus.

Renal Infection
Bacteria. E. coli; Aerobacter aerogenes; Proteus sp; Pseudomonas aeruginosa; Staphylococcus aureus; Streptococcus faecalis; M. tuberculosis.
   Viruses. Coxsackie B; Echo; Mumps; Rubella; Measles.

General infection
Patients with uraemia and immunosuppression are particularly prone to infection and prior to transplantation our patients are screened for Hepatitis Bs antigen and for antibodies against—Hepatitis Bs antigen; Cytomegalovirus; Toxoplasma; Influenza A and B; Herpes.

It is beyond the scope of this work to include details of the serological methods involved in detecting all the above micro-organisms and only the micromethods for detecting streptococcal infection are included here.

STREPTOCOCCAL ANTIBODY TESTS

Streptococci, particularly of Group A β-haemolytic type have been implicated as a frequent cause of acute diffuse proliferative glomerulonephritis. By the time that symptoms such as haematuria occur there may be no obvious evidence of a preceding streptococcal infection.

Several tests have been developed to detect antibodies against streptococcal antigens. Two of the most useful, the antistreptolysin and antihyaluronidase tests are described below and the reader is referred to the DNase B test. Each has particular advantages and routine laboratories favour at least two and sometimes all three. A wider range of tests tends to a higher incidence of positive results.

Antistreptolysin 0 (ASO)

Streptolysin 0 is an oxygen labile haemolysin produced by most strains of Group A streptococci. The principle of the test is that a standard quantity of streptolysin is added to dilutions of the patient's serum and incubated. Where sufficient antistreptolysin is present in the serum the streptolysin is neutralized and erythrocytes added subsequently to the test are not haemolysed. In dilutions where there is insufficient antibody to neutralize the streptolysin, erythrocytes will be haemolysed. The highest dilution showing no haemolysis is the endpoint and is the ASO titre. (Fig. 5.1).

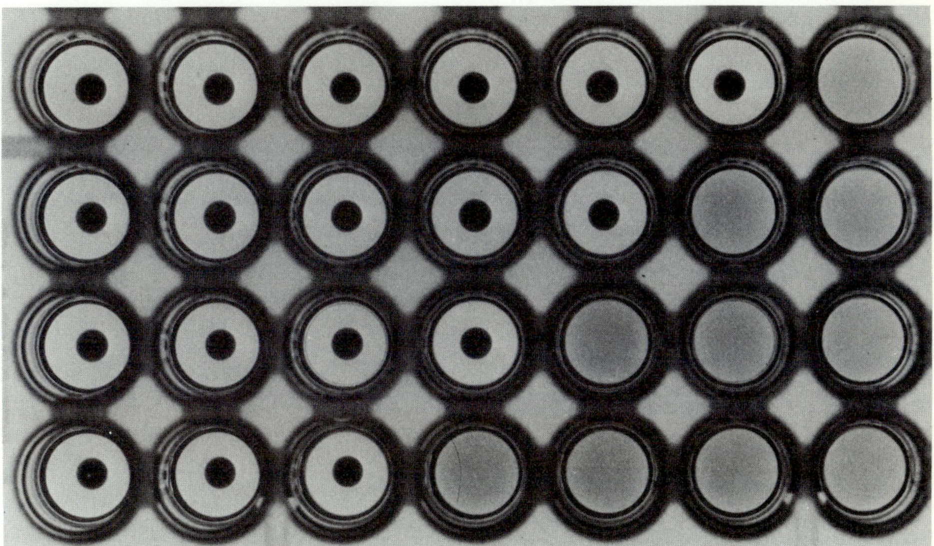

Figure 5.1. Antistreptolysin 0 microtest on two serum samples diluted as in Method (v). The first sample, occupying the top two rows of the plate shows a titre of 1600 and the second sample occupying the bottom two rows of the plate shows a titre of 400.

Equipment
Microtitre plates 12×8 round bottomed wells—$50\,\mu l$ microdiluter, $25\,\mu l$ calibrated dropper pipettes—Microshaker—Microtitre reader—Test tubes 12×75 mm, 14×85 mm—Beaker containing ice.

Reagents
Washed sheep erythrocytes.—Streptolysin 0 reagent.—Streptolysin 0 buffer.—Streptolysin 0 serum standard.

Streptolysin 0 reagent (antigen), buffer and a positive control serum are available commercially and are stored and reconstituted according to the manufacturer's instructions.

Some suppliers enclose instructions for a tube method but the microtitre method below is quicker, more economical and reliable.

Sheep erythrocytes are washed $\times 3$ in saline and resuspended in buffer to give a 2.5% suspension (0.5 ml packed erythrocytes in 19.5 ml buffer).

Collection of specimens
Blood samples are collected under sterile conditions and allowed to clot. Use fresh serum or store frozen until ready for use.

Method
(*i*) Inactivate test sera at 56°C for 30 min and reconstitute streptolysin buffer as directed.

(*ii*) Take two test tubes marked A and B for each patient's test. Prepare a 1 : 20 dilution in A by adding 0.1 ml serum to 1.9 ml ASO buffer and a 1 : 50 dilution in B by adding 0.1 ml serum to 4.9 ml ASO buffer. Mix thoroughly.

(*iii*) Allow two rows of seven wells in the microtitre plate for each serum and mark them A and B. Six wells are required for controls—see below for details. Add two drops (50 μl) of ASO buffer to all test wells.

(*iv*) In row A, add two drops (50 μl) of 1 : 20 serum dilution to the first well. In row B, add two drops (50 μl) of 1 : 50 serum dilution to the first well.

(*v*) Prepare doubling dilutions by transferring 50μl with the microdiluter from well 1 to the next well and continuing along the row.

| Row A: | 40 | 80 | 160 | 320 | 640 | 1280 | 2560 |
| Row B: | 100 | 200 | 400 | 800 | 1600 | 3200 | 6400 |

(*vi*) Reconstitute the streptolysin 0 with cold distilled water (4–6°C). Mix gently but do not shake. Keep streptolysin cold in a beaker of ice water and use within 10 min.

(*vii*) Add one drop (25 μl) of streptolysin 0 reagent to all wells except the erythrocyte control well.

(*viii*) Mix plate on shaker for 15–20 s.

(*ix*) Cover plate with plastic sealing tape to reduce evaporation and incubate at 37°C for 15 min.

(*x*) Add one drop (25 μl) of 2.5% washed sheep erythrocytes to all wells and mix on shaker for 15–20 s to resuspend erythrocytes.

(*xi*) Cover plates and incubate at 37°C for 15 min, mix again to resuspend and incubate at 37°C for a further 30 min.

(*xii*) Allow to settle in the refrigerator at 4°C for $1\frac{1}{2}$–2 h. Read plates over the mirror of the microtitre reader. Even slight haemolysis indicates free streptolysin 0. The end point is the highest dilution giving no haemolysis, only a central red button of erythrocytes in a clear fluid (Fig. 5.1), and is expressed in Todd units.

Controls. The serum standard control requires four wells and the erythrocyte and haemolysin controls one each. Reconstitute the serum standard which represents a 1 : 100 dilution. Serum standard control wells contain:

Well 1	Well 2	Well 3	Well 4
50 μl standard	50 μl standard	50 μl buffer	50 μl buffer
	50 μl buffer	50 μl from well 2	50 μl from well 3
	Mix and transfer	Mix and transfer	Mix and discard
	50 μl to 3.	50 μl to 4.	50 μl.
1 : 100	1 : 200	1 : 400	1 : 800

Complete steps (*vii–xii*) above.
Erythrocyte control well contains: 75 μl buffer; 25 μl sheep erythrocytes.

Haemolysin control well contains: 50 μl buffer; 25 μl streptolysin; 25 μl sheep erythrocytes.

Interpretation
The test must be interpreted in relation to the local community and the general prevalence of streptococcal infections. In general, titres below 100 are not usually significant. The most significant feature is the demonstration of a rising titre in a patient seen first in the early stages of the illness. The ASO titre may rise to a peak by three to five weeks and then gradually falls.

False positive tests can be caused by substances other than antistreptolysin 0 inhibiting the streptolysin, such as serum β lipoproteins found in some liver diseases and certain micro-organisms including pseudomonas and Bacillus cereus.

The test should be repeated if the reference serum does not give the expected titre. The streptolysin control should show complete haemolysis and the erythrocyte control should show no haemolysis.

Antihyaluronidase
Hyaluronidase from Group A streptococci stimulates an antibody response and this can be detected by a neutralization method in which a standard quantity of hyaluronidase is neutralized completely or partially by specific antibody in the patient's serum. Free hyaluronidase can then be assayed by its ability to hydrolyse potassium hyaluronate which otherwise forms a clot in the presence of 2N acetic acid. The clot is more easily visualized if Indian ink has been added to the preparation (Fig. 5.2).

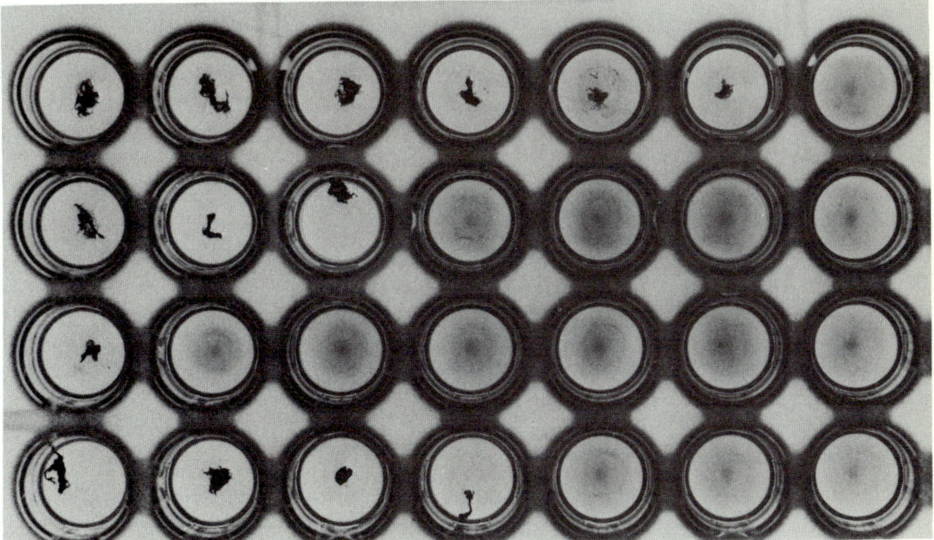

Figure 5.2. Antihyaluronidase microtest on four serum samples, diluted as in Method (iii), showing titres of 1024, 128, 32 and 256. Note how Indian ink has enhanced the visibility of the clot.

Equipment
Microtitre plates, 12×8 round bottomed wells—25 μl microdiluter, 25 μl calibrated dropper pipettes—Microshaker—Microtitre reader—Test tubes (12×75 mm).

Reagents
Hyaluronidase enzyme—Hyaluronidase substrate—Antihyaluronidase serum standard—2N acetic acid—Indian ink—Distilled water.

Commercial kits are available containing hyaluronidase, hyaluronidase substrate and a standard antihyaluronidase control serum (Bacto-AHT, Difco Laboratories).

Method
Test serum should be sterile and refrigerated until use, or used fresh.

(*i*) Prepare a 1 : 16 dilution of each patient's serum in a test tube by adding 1.5 ml of distilled water to 0.1 ml of serum.

(*ii*) Allocate one row of eight wells in the microtitre plate to each test leaving the right hand well free. Add 25 μl of distilled water to each test well, to all but the first of the four standard serum wells and to the enzyme control well. Add 50 μl to the substrate control well.

(*iii*) Add 25 μl of 1 : 16 dilution of patient's test serum to well 1 and prepare doubling dilutions by transferring 25 μl to the next well on the right, mixing and continuing until the 7th well when 25 μl is discarded. The titration range extends from 1 : 32 to 1 : 2048.

(*iv*) Rehydrate the antihyaluronidase serum standard by adding 1 ml of distilled water and dissolve gently by rotating the vial. This is a 1 : 32 dilution. Add 25 μl to wells 1 and 2 of the serum standard control and prepare doubling dilutions to well 4.

Well 1	Well 2	Well 3	Well 4
25 μl standard	25 μl standard	25 μl distilled water	25 μl distilled water
	25 μl distilled water	25 μl from well 2	25 μl from well 3
	Mix and transfer 25 μl to well 3	Mix and transfer 25 μl to well 4	Mix and discard 25 μl
1 : 32	1 : 64	1 : 128	1 : 256

(*v*) Rehydrate the hyaluronidase enzyme by adding 4 ml distilled water and rotating vial to dissolve. Add 25 μl to all wells except the substrate control.

(*vi*) Mix on shaker for 15–20 s, cover plate with plastic sealing tape to prevent evaporation, incubate at 37°C for 15 min and chill at 4°C for 10 min.

(*vii*) While awaiting step (*vi*) to be completed, prepare the Indian ink solution by adding 0.01 ml of Indian ink to 20 ml of distilled water. Rehydrate the hyaluronidase substrate when the primary incubation at 37°C has commenced, by adding 8 ml of the Indian ink solution and dissolve by gentle shaking. Store at 2–10°C and mix periodically. 8 ml of substrate permits 17 tests and one control series.

(*viii*) Add 50 µl of substrate to all wells and mix thoroughly.

(*ix*) Cover and incubate at 37°C for 20 min; chill at 4–10°C for 30 min.

(*x*) Add 25 µl of 2N acetic acid to all wells and mix.

(*xi*) Place plate on the reader and observe wells which contain a clot. The Indian ink is incorporated in the clot and makes it easier to distinguish. In wells having a clot, the fluid is clear while in wells without a clot the fluid is opalescent. The antihyaluronidase titre is the reciprocal of the highest dilution showing clot (Fig. 5.2).

Test wells and antihyaluronidase serum standard wells contain: 25 µl diluted serum; 25 µl enzyme; 50 µl substrate; 25 µl 2N acetic acid.

Controls. Enzyme control well contains: 25 µl distilled water; 25 µl enzyme; 50 µl substrate; 25 µl 2N acetic acid. Substrate control well contains: 50 µl distilled water; 50 µl substrate; 25 µl 2N acetic acid. The enzyme control contains no antihyaluronidase and should show no clot. The substrate control contains substrate but no enzyme and should show clot formation. The reference antihyaluronidase serum standard should show the correct titre.

Interpretation

Not all patients respond to streptococcal infection by producing a significant antihyaluronidase titre. Hence a negative result does not exclude streptococcal infection. This test is used to supplement the antistreptolysin 0 test and may be positive where the ASO was not significant. Normal titres again depend on the particular population but titres up to 256 may not indicate infection. As with the ASO test, a rising titre demonstrated over three to five weeks is more significant than a single elevated determination.

Antideoxyribonuclease B

Streptococci produce several deoxyribonucleases (DNases) but DNaseB is confined largely to Group A β-haemolytic streptococci and is the DNase of choice in detecting infections by this group.

The anti-DNaseB test is considered by some authorities to be the test of choice in detecting streptococcal infections but has not been widely used. It is positive in situations where antistreptolysin is negative and is particularly useful in cases where skin infections have occurred and have been followed by glomerulonephritis. Test kits are available commercially and technical details are given by Klein (1976).

ANTINUCLEAR ANTIBODIES

The group of autoantibodies found most commonly in patients with renal disease are those detected in patients with systemic lupus erythematosus. Antinuclear antibodies (ANA) occur at some stage in all patients with systemic lupus and their presence indicates consideration of the possibility of renal involvement or may provide confirmatory evidence if a renal biopsy is suggestive of lupus nephritis. ANA are detected by immunofluorescence and by DNA-binding radioimmunoassays.

Immunofluorescence

Equipment
Cryostat—Clean microscope slides and coverslips—Moist chamber—Fluorescence microscope—Marker pen—Forceps—Container for freezing mixture.

Reagents
Freezing mixture, e.g. liquid nitrogen–isopentane slurry.

Phosphate-buffered saline, 0.1M phosphate, pH 7.1: NaCl 8.5g; Na_2HPO_4 1.07g; $NaH_2PO_4.2H_2O$ 0.39g. Make up to 1 litre with distilled water.

Veronal buffer, pH 8.6: sodium veronal 10.3g; NaCl 6.2g. Adjust pH to 8.6 with HCl. Make up to 1 litre with distilled water.

Buffered glycerol mountant. Mix equal volumes of A.R. glycerol and the veronal buffer.

Antiserum. Polyvalent antihuman immunoglobulin serum labelled with FITC.

Method
(*i*) Snap-freeze a block of mouse liver either alone or as part of a composite block containing all or some of the following—mouse stomach, rat kidney, pig adrenal and human thyroid. The composite block permits the most economical use of materials and labour in screening for a spectrum of autoantibodies.

(*ii*) Cut 4–6 μm sections in a cryostat and mount two sections on each slide.

(*iii*) Dry sections with a fan for 2 h at room temperature or overnight at 4°C.

(*iv*) Draw a circle on the undersurface of the slide around the outline of each section with a marking pen or diamond marker to identify the region where reagents and coverslip are to be applied.

(*v*) Prepare a 1 : 5 dilution of the patient's serum in PBS (pH 7.1) and apply a drop to the section.

(*vi*) Place slides in a moist chamber, cover to prevent evaporation and leave for 30 min. The plastic tray with a gel foam base (Nairn, 1976) is very suitable.

(*vii*) Wash off serum and give two 5 min washes in PBS.

(*viii*) Dry around sections and apply a drop of FITC anti-human globulin.

(*ix*) Leave in the closed moist chamber for 30 min.

(*x*) Rinse off FITC antiserum and wash twice for 5 min in PBS.

(*xi*) Mount coverslip over each section using the buffered glycerol mountant. Controls should include a positive serum, a negative serum and FITC antiglobulin alone.

Patterns of nuclear staining
A peripheral staining pattern is produced by sera with antibodies against double-stranded DNA.

A diffuse or homogeneous pattern of staining is associated with antibodies to deoxyribonucleoprotein.

A speckled pattern is produced by antibodies against certain of the soluble or extractable nuclear antigens, including ribonucleoprotein and the Sm antigen. These antibodies can also be detected by haemagglutination, complement fixation and immunodiffusion (Akizuki et al, 1977).

Nucleolar antibodies may also be detected and are commonly associated with scleroderma.

The fluorescent patterns of staining should be observed and titres may be determined for positive sera. The incidence of ANA increases with age in the general population and titres up to 1 : 16 or 1 : 32 may be found in apparently normal individuals.

Crithidia luciliae

A fluorescent antibody test using the haemaflagellate *Crithidia luciliae* kinetoplast as a double-stranded DNA substrate has received favourable recognition. (Sontheimer & Gilliam, 1978). The kinetoplast is a modified mitochondrion containing a localized collection of double-stranded DNA. This method necessitates the maintenance of cultures which must be kept free of bacterial and fungal contamination and should be harvested in the log phase of growth. The kinetoplast is a rather small body which should not be confused with other staining areas including the nucleus and a spot at the flagellar base.

Lymphocytes in metaphase

A further method for DNA antibodies includes using cultured human lymphocytes, in which cell division has been held in metaphase, as the substrate for a fluorescent antibody test (Somerfield, personal communication).

DNA binding

The DNA binding assay is a sensitive method of measuring antibodies against double-stranded DNA which appear to be those most closely associated with the clinical features of systemic lupus erythematosus and the development of nephritis.

The principle of this test is that ^{125}I labelled DNA combines with ANA in the patient's serum and is then precipitated by saturated ammonium sulphate. The ^{125}I in the precipitate is then assayed by scintillation counter and is a measure of the ANA in the patient's serum. A reference curve is drawn of counts against units/ml from four standards of known ANA concentration and a buffer, which is the zero point on the curve. Sera are first incubated at 56°C for 30 min to eliminate nonspecific binding to DNA by some proteins. All tests are performed in duplicate and the mean values are used for plotting the reference curve and estimation of unknown antibody levels.

Up to 25 units of activity are found in normal individuals but the precise diagnostic level should be determined for each laboratory. Kits containing all reagents and suitable tubes for the test are available commercially (Radiochemical Centre, Amersham, England).

This is a well standardized test which is straightforward to perform. It is usual to screen for ANA using an immunofluorescence test and then to proceed to DNA binding in selected cases. An intervening test with *Crithidia luciliae* or lymphocytes in metaphase may be a further basis of selection for antibodies against double-stranded DNA.

Comment on ANA
Serum ANA are found not only in patients with systemic lupus erythematosus but also in rheumatoid arthritis, scleroderma, mixed connective tissue disease, some normal individuals, and from time to time in other conditions. They may also be induced by drugs. Under these circumstances the precise type of ANA and its titre may become important in diagnosis and in monitoring progression of the disease.

Antibodies against double-stranded DNA appear to be the most specific antibody for systemic lupus erythematosus and to correlate in a general way with disease activity. Patients in remission may develop weaker ANA fluorescent tests and show a reduction in DNA binding. ANA induced by drugs, with the exception of hydrallazine, are not usually associated with DNA binding activity.

It is of some interest that patients in chronic renal failure, and those on chronic dialysis develop antibodies against nuclear antigens, particularly extractable nuclear antigens but pathological effects have not been attributed to them (Nolph et al, 1978).

ANTIGLOMERULAR BASEMENT MEMBRANE ANTIBODIES

High levels of antibodies directed against glomerular basement membrane in serum of patients with Goodpasture's syndrome, can be detected on frozen sections of normal human kidney by the indirect immunofluorescence staining technique described earlier for the detection of ANA. Preliminary trials should be conducted with a variety of human kidneys so that one can be obtained which has a low level of background glomerular staining from globulin within the capillary walls. A few laboratories have developed sensitive radioimmuno-assay procedures to monitor basement membrane antibody levels and these are of assistance in assessing the effects of treatment, particularly plasmapheresis on the circulating antibody level.

ANTITUBULAR BASEMENT MEMBRANE ANTIBODIES

Serum antibodies reacting with renal tubular basement membrane are found in some patients with Goodpasture's syndrome and may occur in interstitial nephritis particularly if due to methicillin hypersensitivity. They may also occur in renal graft rejection.

ANTITUBULAR BRUSH BORDER ANTIBODIES

Although these antibodies have been identified in experimental autologous immune complex nephritis, isolated reports of clinical examples await confirmation. Such antibodies must be distinguished from heterologous antibody in human serum which cross-reacts with gastric parietal cells and the renal tubular brush border of rats (Ireton et al, 1971).

OTHER AUTOANTIBODIES

It is surprising that the only common autoantibody apart from ANA to be implicated in immune complex renal disease has been the thyroglobulin antibody which has been reported as a complication of radio-iodine therapy (Ploth et al, 1978).

Antibodies directed against cells lining the loop of Henle have been detected in serum but have not been associated consistently with renal disease, although one patient had a defect of renal tubular acidification (Chanarin et al, 1974).

TAMM-HORSFALL PROTEIN ANTIBODIES

Tamm-Horsfall glycoprotein is secreted by the ascending limb of the loop of Henle and distal convoluted tubule. It has been suggested that damage to this portion of the tubule, such as might occur in reflux nephropathy as a consequence of vesico-ureteric urinary reflux, could result in the release of Tamm-Horsfall protein into the renal interstitial tissue and blood stream and might provoke an immunological reaction. However Fasth et al (1977) were unable to show a correlation between antibody titres and the presence of vesico-ureteric reflux or kidney scarring, but have recently shown further elevation of titres in acute pyelonephritis if reflux is present.

REFERENCES

Akizuki M, Powers R, Holman H R 1977 Comparative study of immunologic methods for demonstration of antibodies to soluble nuclear antigens. Immunofluorescence, haemagglutination, complement fixation, and immunodiffusion. Arthritis and Rheumatism 20: 693–701

Chanarin I, Loewi G, Tavill A S, Swain C P, Tidmarsh E 1974 Defect of renal tubular acidification with antibody to loop of Henle. Lancet 2: 317–318

Fasth A, Hanson L Å, Asscher A W 1977 Autoantibodies to Tamm-Horsfall protein in detection of vesicoureteric reflux and kidney scarring. Archives of Disease in Childhood 52: 560–562

Ireton H J C, Muller H K, McGiven A R 1971 Human antibody against rat gastric parietal cells and kidney brush border. Clinical and Experimental Immunology 8: 783–789

Klein G C 1976 Immune response to streptococcal infection. In: Manual of Clinical Immunology ed Rose N R, Friedman H ch 33 American Society for Microbiology, Washington

Nairn R C 1976 Fluorescent Protein Tracing, 4th edn. Churchill Livingstone, Edinburgh

Nolph K D, Ghods A J, Sharp G C, Siemsen A W 1978 Antibodies to nuclear antigens in patients with renal failure. Journal of Laboratory and Clinical Medicine 91: 559–567

Ploth D W, Fitz A, Schnetzler D, Seidenfeld J, Wilson C B 1978 Thyroglobulin-anti-thyroglobulin immune complex glomerulonephritis complicating radioiodine therapy. Clinical Immunology and Immunopathology 9: 327–334

Sontheimer R D, Gilliam J N 1978 An immunofluorescence assay for double-stranded DNA antibodies using the Crithidia luciliae kinetoblast as a double-stranded DNA substrate. Journal of Laboratory and Clinical Medicine 91: 550–558

6
Urine

C. M. Andre, A. R. McGiven and Susan M. McQuilkan

The examination of urine continues to play an important role in the investigation of patients with renal disease. The application of physico-chemical and immunological methods has enabled the clinician to gather useful diagnostic information in a wide spectrum of renal disorders including glomerulonephritis, pyelonephritis, graft rejection and multiple myeloma.

PROTEINURIA

Normal urine contains a small amount of protein, usually less than 0.25 g/day. Approximately two thirds of this protein is derived from plasma and one third from the secretions of the kidney and urogenital tract. Well over 30 plasma protein constituents have been identified in the urine, most of these occurring in trace amounts. A glycoprotein known as Tamm-Horsfall glycoprotein accounts for the majority of the non-plasma protein constituents in urine.

Increased loss of proteins in urine, proteinuria, has been recognized as a cardinal sign of renal disease for well over a century now and whenever detected requires an explanation or merits investigation for an underlying cause. From a practical standpoint proteinuria may be considered according to the following classification.

Overflow proteinuria
This type of proteinuria is due to the presence of abnormal quantities of low molecular weight proteins in plasma. These low molecular weight proteins are filtered to a variable extent across the glomerulus and saturate the tubular re-absorptive process. This type of proteinuria is exemplified by Bence-Jones proteinuria, myoglobinuria and the excretion of lysozyme.

Glomerular proteinuria
This is characterized by the abnormal excretion of proteins of molecular weight greater than 60 000 due to some abnormality of glomerular structure or function. The quantity of protein excreted may vary from less than one to more than 30 g/d. The proteinuria may be selective or nonselective.

Excessive glomerular protein losses result in a typical plasma protein pattern namely low levels of albumin and commonly IgG, normal or low levels of α1 globulins and an increase of high molecular weight proteins, α2 macroglobulin, fibrinogen, β lipoprotein and often IgM.

Tubular proteinuria
This type is characterized by the loss of proteins of molecular weights less than 70 000. It is readily identified by sodium dodecyl sulphate polyacrylamide gel electrophoresis or by measuring β2 microglobulin excretion. It should however be noted that if the glomerular filtration rate is considerably impaired nearly all patients will excrete increased amounts of filtered small molecular weight proteins due to the increased plasma levels and consequent saturation of, or concurrent damage to, the reabsorptive tubular process of the remaining functioning nephrons.

Nephrogenic proteinuria
This type of proteinuria may be caused by increased secretion of specific proteins into the tubular fluid and to the loss of structural proteins from the nephrons.

Important variations in the excretion rate of the main glycoprotein secreted in urine, Tamm-Horsfall glycoprotein, have yet to be demonstrated but it is a major constituent of casts. Losses of structural proteins of the nephrons have been described both for basement membrane like material and for tubular elements but have yet to be specifically related to clinical syndromes.

INVESTIGATION OF URINE PROTEINS

The quantitation of proteinuria is a useful aid in assessing the presence and severity of many renal disorders and in monitoring their progress. In addition this permits the urine to be concentrated to an optimal protein concentration for further analyses by electrophoresis or immunoelectrophoresis. Appropriate specific protein analyses as described in the following techniques, both qualitative and quantitative, may provide further diagnostic information.

Estimation of total protein in urine
The urinary proteins are precipitated by cold ethanolic phosphotungstic acid. The protein precipitate is separated by centrifugation and washed with ethanol. The precipitate is then redissolved in biuret reagent. The colour which develops is compared with protein standards. A correction for the urine blank is included.

Specimen
A 24 h specimen of urine is stored in a refrigerator at 4°C during the collection period and until time for analysis. Analyse fresh, if not store aliquots frozen. Heavily infected urines are unsuitable.

Reagents
(*i*) *Ethanolic phosphotungstic acid.* Add 100 ml concentrated HCl (SG 1.18) to 200 ml distilled water. Cool. Add to this mixture 1463 ml 99.7–100% (v/v) ethanol. Add 30 g phosphotungstic acid and dissolve. Filter and store at 4°C. The reagent is stable for at least two months.

(*ii*) *95% (v/v) absolute ethanol.*

(*iii*) *Biuret reagent and blank biuret reagent.* The same reagent and storage conditions as used for the estimation of serum total protein. *See* Total Protein Quantitation in Chapter 2.

(*iv*) *NaCl solution.* Dissolve 9 g NaCl in 1 litre distilled water.

(*v*) *Protein standards.* 0.2 g/l, 2 g/l. The protein concentration of a secondary standard which is fresh human serum from a normal pool is standardized against the 'standard reference material' used for primary standardization of the serum total protein assay. The biuret procedure for this standardization is the same as detailed in Chapter 2. The serum pool is then appropriately diluted with NaCl solution to give 0.2 g/l and 2 g/l secondary standards. The stock serum pool is stored frozen and the working standards are prepared weekly from this and stored at 4°C. Preservation with azide is not recommended because of its instability in acid conditions.

(*vi*) *Quality control.* Commercial urine controls are available.

Method

(*i*) Into test tubes pipette centrifuged urine, quality control sample and protein standards as follows—

	Test	Blank
Urine or appropriate dilution	2 ml	2 ml
Quality control sample	2 ml	2 ml
Protein standard 0.2 g/l	2 ml	2 ml
Protein standard 2 g/l	2 ml	2 ml

(*ii*) To each test tube add 8 ml cold ethanolic phosphotungstic acid.

(*iii*) Mix by inversion and stand in refrigerator (4°C) for at least 5 min.

(*iv*) Centrifuge at 1000 g for 5 min.

(*v*) Decant the supernatant removing last drops by absorption on filter paper.

(*vi*) Add 1 ml absolute ethanol to all tubes, disperse the protein pellets by means of a mechanical mixer, centrifuge the tubes at 1000 g for 5 min, decant the ethanol and again remove residual fluid on filter paper.

(*vii*) To each blank tube add 5 ml biuret blank reagent and to each test add 5 ml biuret reagent.

(*viii*) Dissolve the precipitates using a vortex mixer and then stand tubes for 30 min.

(*ix*) Inspect tubes to ensure that the reaction mixtures are free of particulate matter, if not clear by centrifugation.

(*x*) Measure the absorbance (A) of the biuret reagent, *i.e.* reagent blank and tests at 540 nm in 10 mm cuvettes with distilled water as reference. Measure the absorbance of the blanks at the same wavelength with the blank biuret reagent as reference.

Calculation

$$\frac{\text{(A) sample test} - \text{(A) reagent blank} + \text{sample blank}}{\text{(A) standard test} - \text{(A) reagent blank} + \text{standard blank}} \times 0.2 \text{ or } 2.0 = \text{g/l}$$

Report results in g/d.

Reference range

In healthy adults the daily urinary protein excretion is believed to be less than 0.25 g. It should be noted that there are a number of factors which affect the excretion of urine proteins thus each laboratory should determine its own reference range.

Each laboratory should regularly check that Beer's law is obeyed by setting up a series of standards within the range of 0.2 g/l to 5 g/l.

It should be realized that the ethanolic phosphotungstic acid precipitating agent will precipitate Tamm-Horsfall glycoprotein, which is the most abundant of the proteins derived from the urinary tract itself, as well as urinary proteins that originate from plasma. Other precipitating acid reagents have been used, *e.g.* perchloric and sulphosalicylic acid. The precipitant used has a major influence on the qualitative and quantitative recovery of proteins from urine. The method could be used with trichloroacetic acid as a substitute for the ethanolic phosphotungstic acid. However, certain glycoproteins are soluble in 5–10% trichloroacetic acid.

Quantitative investigation of urine proteins

Selectivity of proteinuria

Differential protein clearances are of value in predicting the effect of steroid or cyclophosphamide therapy of nephrotic patients with selective proteinuria, even when proliferative glomerular lesions are present. The renal clearance of a lower molecular weight protein such as albumin or transferrin is compared with a higher molecular weight protein, *e.g.* IgG. Albumin, transferrin, IgG and $\alpha 2$ macroglobulin have been variously used to determine the selectivity of proteinurias.

Procedure

(*i*) *Samples.* A serum sample is taken concurrently with a timed or random urine sample.

(*ii*) *Quantitation of selected proteins.* Transferrin and IgG concentrations are determined in duplicate on both urine and serum samples by electro-immunoassay—prior concentration of the urine sample is not necessary. *N.B.* The IgG molecule is not carbamylated, resulting in anodic-cathodic immuno-precipitates. *See* Electroimmunoassay in Chapter 2. Electrophoresis of urine and serum samples before quantitation acts as a valuable reference for assessing the required dilutions for electroimmunoassay and visual interpretation.

(*iii*) *The clearance ratio* of IgG to transferrin is determined from:

$$\text{IgG/transferrin clearance ratio} = \frac{\text{urine IgG g/l}}{\text{serum IgG g/l}} \div \frac{\text{urine transferrin g/l}}{\text{serum transferrin g/l}}$$

Limitations of protein clearance ratios

Circulating low molecular weight breakdown products, *e.g.* immunoglobulin fragments, will result in erroneous immunochemical quantitation, and indicate high renal clearances. Another anomaly is that renal clearance of proteins is not solely dependent on their molecular weights.

This test is of limited value in predicting the type of histological lesion in glomeruli, although in nephrotic children, a highly selective proteinuria suggests the minimal change lesion.

Interpretation
There are various ways of expressing the renal clearance of proteins depending on the number of specific proteins quantitated. However, for practical purposes, the IgG/transferrin clearance ratio is considered to provide sufficient information on which to predict a response to steroid therapy.

An IgG/transferrin clearance ratio of less than 0.2 indicates a selective proteinuria likely to respond to therapy.

An IgG/transferrin clearance ratio of greater than 0.3 indicates a proteinuria of low selectivity.

The value of protein clearance studies in the detection and prediction of renal allograft rejection is referred to in Chapter 8.

Qualitative investigation of urine proteins

Electrophoresis of urine is used in the investigation of proteinuria, in particular for the demonstration of Bence-Jones protein. An early morning urine sample is adequate for the qualitative investigation of urine, and of less inconvenience to the patient than a 24 h collection.

Total protein
It is necessary to quantitate the urine protein in order to ascertain the degree of concentration required. *See* Estimation of Total Protein in Urine.

Concentration of urine
Before electrophoresis and immunoelectrophoresis, a urine sample should be concentrated to give 25 g protein/l. There are several methods available for concentrating urines. The Minicon—B 15 Concentrator (Amicon Corporation) is simple, quick and satisfactory. It is a disposable, multiple ultra filter which requires no support equipment and can be operated unattended. The inner surface of each of the eight separate chambers consists of a selective permeable membrane with a molecular retention of 15 000 daltons. This membrane is backed in turn with wick pads to absorb water and permeating molecules below 15 000 daltons. Retained macrosolutes are progressively concentrated as the volume of samples in the chamber diminishes. Graduation lines at $\times 5$, $\times 10$, $\times 25$, $\times 50$, $\times 100$ indicate concentration ratios.

Procedure. Filter urine sample through Whatman No. 1 filter paper. (The Minicon chamber holds 5 ml). Determine the required concentration factor from the initial protein concentration. Fill chamber through small hole by means of a Pasteur pipette. Care should be taken to avoid scratching the membrane or exceeding the fill line. When the desired concentration level is reached, the concentrate is recovered by inserting a Pasteur pipette to the bottom of the chamber. Although the absorbent capacity of each chamber is about three times the sample volume, the re-use of chambers in which abnormal urines have been concentrated is not recommended. Store Minicon-B 15 Concentrator at 4°C when not in use.

Electrophoresis
Ideally a urine concentrate should be electrophoresed alongside the patient's serum, thus allowing the investigator to utilize clearance concepts in the interpretation of the electrophoretic patterns. A control serum sample must be used to enable position identification of the various protein fractions. The procedure for the electrophoresis of urine is similar to that used for serum. *See* Agarose Gel Electrophoresis in Chapter 2. *N.B.* The urine concentrate is not diluted with the glycerol-tris-veronal diluent before electrophoresis.

Immunoelectrophoresis
Immunoelectrophoresis enables protein fractions revealed by electrophoresis of the urine concentrate to be identified. It will confirm the presence of monoclonal light chains, *i.e.* Bence-Jones protein, as well as monoclonal immunoglobulins and/or their fragments.

The procedure for characterizing separated protein fractions in urine is similar to that for serum. *See* Qualitative Immunoelectrophoresis in Chapter 2.

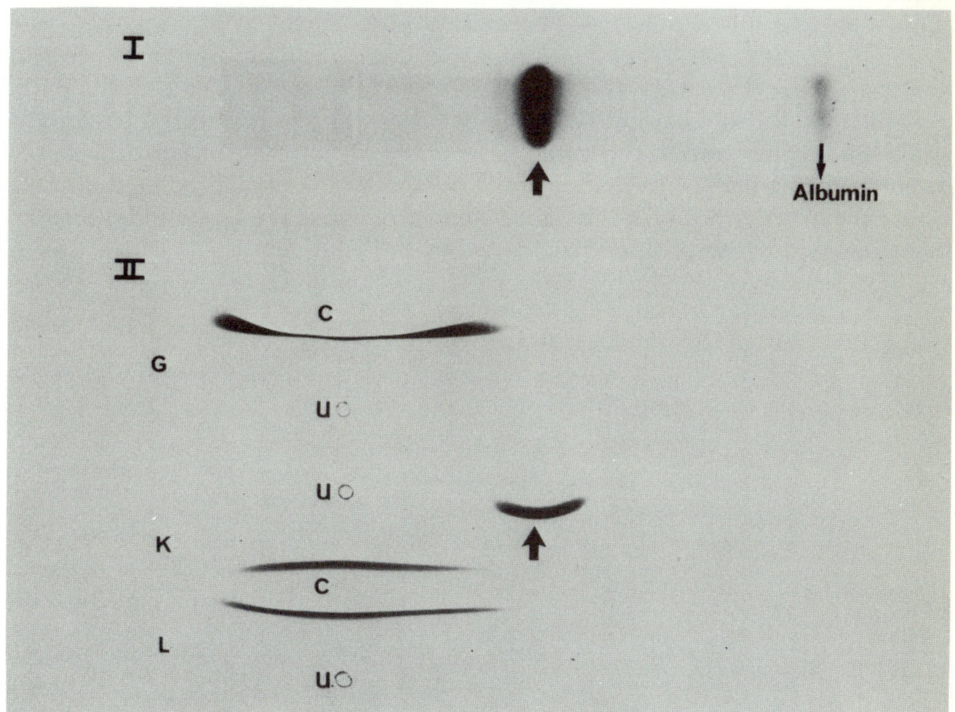

Figure 6.1. An abnormal discrete band is arrowed on the urine electrophoretogram, I. The immunoelectrophoretogram, II, shows abnormal bowing of the kappa arc, arrowed, corresponding in position to the abnormal band in I.
Note. The monoclonal immunoglobulin present in the patient's serum was IgG, hence the use of antiserum to IgG to exclude the presence of the same immunoglobulin in the urine.
G=anti-IgG trough   K= antikappa   L=antilambda   U=urine sample   C=control serum well

Interpretation
It cannot be overstressed that in order to confirm Bence-Jones proteinuria, a discrete band which indicates its monoclonal nature must be seen on electrophoresis (Fig. 6.1). More than one abnormal discrete band is not uncommon and it is therefore essential that the abnormal configuration visualized immunoelectrophoretically lines up with the discrete band detected on electrophoresis.

Molecular weight analysis of urine proteins by polyacrylamide gel-sodium dodecyl sulphate electrophoresis

Polyacrylamide gel electrophoresis in the presence of sodium dodecyl sulphate (SDS) separates proteins or polypeptides on the basis of their molecular weight. The negatively charged detergent ions bind to the protein and the amount bound depends on the size of the protein. This swamps the charge of the native protein thus giving all proteins a similar charge density. Electrophoresis in polyacrylamide then sieves the proteins and separates them according to size, their relative mobility being inversely proportional to the molecular weight. By comparing the mobility of a protein with proteins of known molecular weight it is possible to determine its size.

Equipment
Direct current power supply—Thermostatically controlled water bath.

Electrophoresis tank. This consists of two vessels which form an upper and lower chamber (Fig. 6.2). The upper chamber has holes drilled into the base, in which the gel tubes are fitted by rubber grommets to maintain a watertight seal. Both upper and lower tanks have platinum wire electrodes, the lower chamber being the positive electrode. The upper tank should be held directly above the lower tank so that electrical contact between the liquid in both tanks is maintained via the polyacrylamide gel in the glass tubes.

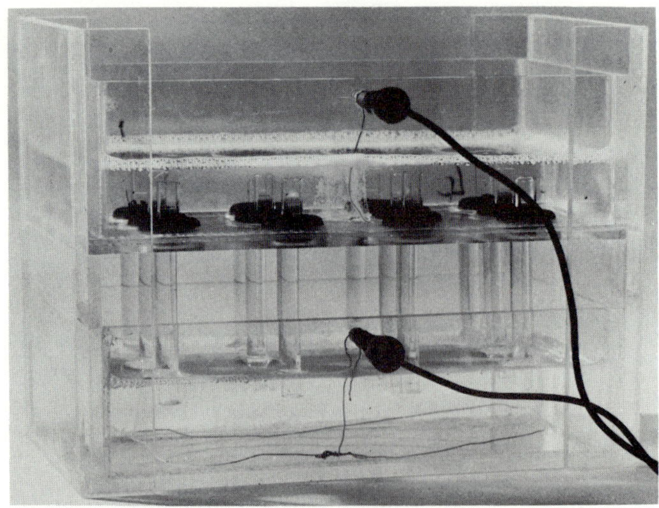

Figure 6.2. Apparatus for polyacrylamide gel electrophoresis.

Glass tubes for polyacrylamide gels have an internal diameter of 6 mm and are 75 mm in length and should fit firmly into the rubber grommets of the upper electrophoresis chamber. The tubes must be scrupulously cleaned and dried before use.

Other items are Büchner 100 ml flask—Measuring cylinders: 25 ml; 10 ml × 2—Syringes: 20 ml with 18 gauge needle or small bore teflon tubing for rapid pouring of polyacrylamide gels; 20 ml with 22 gauge needle 80 mm long for extracting gels from the glass tube—Test tubes, 15 × 120 mm—Scalpel blades—Parafilm.

Reagents

(*i*) *Acrylamide stock solution.* 22.2 g acrylamide; 0.6 g N, N-methylene bis-acrylamide; dissolve in distilled water and make up to 100 ml. Filter and keep at 4°C in a dark bottle. The solution is stable for months but should be filtered before use.

(*ii*) *Electrophoresis buffer.* 0.2M phosphate buffer pH 7.2; 7.8 g $NaH_2PO_4.H_2O$; 38.6 g $Na_2HPO_4.7H_2O$; 2 g sodium dodecyl sulphate (SDS). Dissolve in distilled water and make up to 1 litre.

(*iii*) *Incubation buffer.* 0.01M phosphate buffer containing approximately 10 g/l SDS. The electrophoresis buffer is diluted 1 : 20 with an aqueous solution of SDS, 10 g/l.

(*iv*) *Marker dye.* 1 g/l aqueous Bromphenol Blue.

(*v*) *Staining solution.* 250 ml isopropanol; 100 ml acetic acid; 1 g Coomassie Brilliant Blue R-250. Make up to 1 litre with distilled water.

(*vi*) *Destaining solution.* 100 ml acetic acid; 100 ml methanol. Make up to 1 litre with distilled water.

(*vii*) *Other reagents.* Glycerol, 2-mercaptoethanol, N, N, N′, N′-tetramethyl-ethyldiamine (TEMED), ammonium persulphate AR grade.

(*viii*) *Standard protein solution.* A mixture of proteins of known molecular weight, each at a concentration of 1 g/l, is prepared in the incubation buffer. *e.g.* IgG (mol. wt. 150 000), albumin (mol. wt. 68 000), ovalbumin (mol. wt. 43 000), carbonic anhydrase (mol. wt. 29 000), haemoglobin (mol. wt. 16 000). Aliquots of 5 μl of the protein mixture may be stored frozen until required.

Method

An aliquot of a 24 h urine sample is clarified by centrifugation and concentrated to 1 g protein/l as described previously. 50 μl of the concentrate is used for analysis.

Preparation of samples for electrophoresis. To the standard protein mixture (5 μl) and the urine concentrate (50 μl) add 50 μl of the 0.01M phosphate buffer containing 10 g/l SDS. Incubate all the samples at 50–60°C in a water bath for 30–60 min, then to each sample add one drop of glycerol to facilitate sample application and add 5 μl of the marker dye. Mix thoroughly.

Preparation of 70 g/l gels. Before preparing the gels, seal one end of each 6 × 75 mm glass tube with parafilm and support the tubes vertically. The grommets of the upper electrophoresis chamber make an excellent tube holder for gel pouring. The following recipe is sufficient for making 12 gels—

15 ml 0.2M phosphate buffer, 9.5 ml filtered stock acrylamide and 4 ml distilled water are placed in the Büchner flask and deaerated. The solution is cooled on ice and 1.5 ml of freshly prepared aqueous ammonium persulphate solution 1.5 g/1 and 40 μl of TEMED are added. After gentle mixing, the solution is poured quickly and carefully into the tubes with a 20 ml syringe with a teflon tube outlet. Ensure that air bubbles are excluded and each tube is filled to within 5 to 10 mm of the top. After pouring the gels, carefully layer a few drops of distilled water on top of the gel solution. Allow the gels to polymerize undisturbed. This takes between 30 to 60 min. Polymerization is complete when a sharp interface is formed between the gel and water layer.

N.B. All equipment used to pour the gels must be washed with water before polymerization occurs to facilitate their reuse. Remove the parafilm seal and insert the tubes into the rubber grommets of the electrophoresis chamber if not already done. The incompletely filled end of the tube protrudes into the upper chamber so that the interface between gel and aqueous layer is visible. Fill the upper and lower electrophoresis chambers with 0.2M phosphate buffer diluted 1 : 1 with distilled water. Ensure that there are no leaks where the tubes fit into the grommets and that all the tubes are immersed to a depth of 5 to 10 mm in buffer in the lower chamber. Connect the apparatus to the power pack, remembering that the positive electrode is connected to the lower chamber. Switch on the power to a constant current of 8–10 mA/gel, *i.e.* for 12 gels the current should be about 100 mA and the voltage less than 50 V. Electrophoresis is carried out for 10 min before applying the samples. This removes unwanted ionic species from the gels and is a check on the system.

Application of sample. Switch off the current to the electrophoretic chambers and carefully layer the samples on top of the gels using a Pasteur pipette. This operation is easily performed with a little practice. The samples being heavier than the phosphate buffer readily settle on top of the gels.

Electrophoresis. Electrophoresis is performed with a constant current of 8–10 mA/gel until the marker dye is at a distance of 5 mm from the lower end of the gel. This takes approximately 4 h. After electrophoresis switch off the current and remove the tubes from the grommets. The gels are eased out of the tubes by very gently squirting electrophoresis buffer, using a syringe fitted with a long needle, 22 gauge × 80 mm, between the gel and glass tube. The needle can be eased further and further down the tube and by gentle rotation of the tube the gel should free from the glass and be extracted when the needle is withdrawn. Mark the position of the tracking dye by nicking the gel with a scalpel blade.

Staining and destaining. Transfer the gels to suitable test tubes containing the Coomassie Blue staining solution and leave to soak overnight. Alternatively the gels may be rapidly stained by placing the test tubes in a 60°C water bath for 2 h. After staining the Coomassie Blue is decanted and replaced with destaining solution. Unbound dye is removed by heating in a 60°C water bath and changing the destaining solution several times. Adequate destaining may take four or more hours to achieve.

Interpretation of results

Compare the test gels with the standard gel. Observe the molecular weight pattern of the proteins in the test gels. A tubular proteinuria is characterized by the presence of proteins of molecular weights less than 70 000 whereas the presence of proteins of molecular weight greater than 60 000 indicates a glomerular proteinuria. In cases of marked renal impairment the whole spectrum of molecular weight proteins may be seen (Fig. 6.3). It should be noted that proteins which exist in polymeric forms, *e.g.* albumin may be seen on SDS polyacrylamide gel electrophoresis as multiple bands.

Alternatively measure the migration distance of each protein band in the standard gel and divide by the migration distance of the marker dye. This gives the relative mobility of each protein band. Plot the mobilities of the standard proteins against the logarithm of their respective molecular weight. The graph should be a straight line. Determine the molecular weights of the urinary proteins by measuring their relative mobilities and interpolating on the graph. A semiquantitative measure of the protein fractions may be obtained by densitometry.

Proteins containing intra-chain disulphide bonds which restrict the amount of SDS binding may have relative mobilities which lead to inaccurate estimates of their molecular weights. The relative mobility of albumin and other proteins which contain intra-chain disulphide bonds, are more reliably measured after

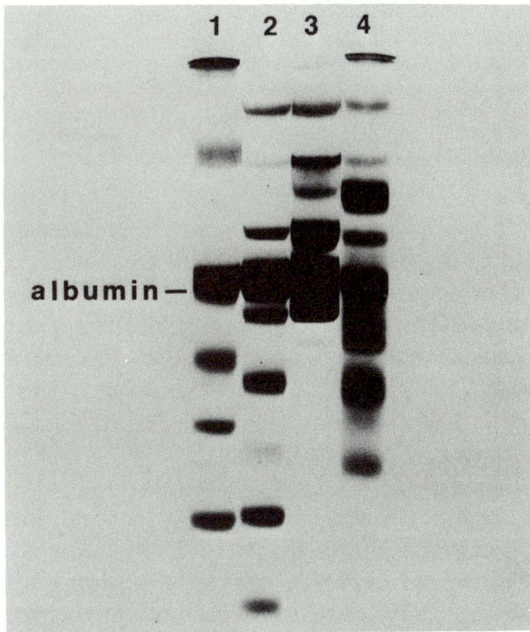

Figure 6.3. SDS polyacrylamide gel electrophoretogram of standard proteins, 1 and urine concentrates 2, 3 and 4. The origin is at the top of the figure and the migration of proteins is in descending order according to their molecular weights. The position of albumin, 68 000 molecular weight is indicated in the standard gel, 1. In gel 2, there is a predominance of lower molecular weight proteins, whilst higher molecular weight proteins are seen in gel 3. A range of both higher and lower molecular weight proteins is seen in gel 4.

prior reduction with mercaptoethanol. This reduction results in increased SDS binding. The presence of mercaptoethanol in the standard protein mixture will also partially reduce immunoglobulin disulphide bonds and liberate heavy and light chains (Fig. 6.4).

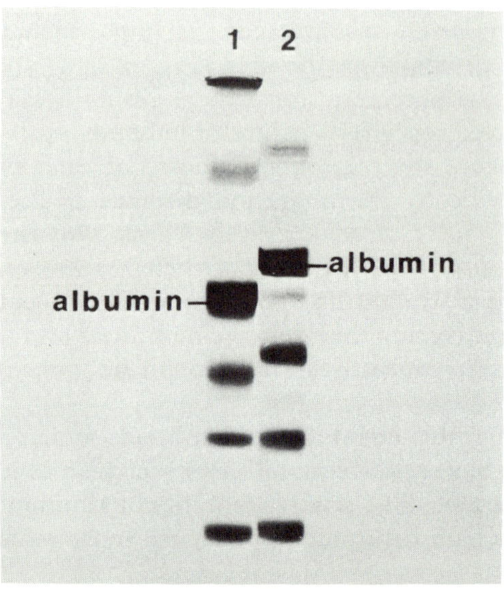

Figure 6.4. SDS polyacrylamide electrophoretogram of standard proteins with and without mercaptoethanol. The very high molecular weight protein band at the origin (top) of gel 1, is aggregated IgG. The standard proteins in descending order of molecular weight are IgG, albumin, ovalbumin, carbonic anhydrase and haemoglobin chains. In the presence of mercaptoethanol, gel 2, the mobility of the major protein bands on either side of albumin has been retarded relative to the proteins in gel 1 which was run without mercaptoethanol. The smaller band below albumin in gel 2 is the heavy chain component liberated by the reduction of IgG by mercaptoethanol.

To prepare a standard protein mixture containing mercaptoethanol add 5 μl of mercaptoethanol to the protein standard and treat as previously described.

Technical note. If polymerization of acrylamide occurs too slowly or not at all increase the amount of TEMED and/or ammonium persulphate.

N.B. Unpolymerized acrylamide is a neurotoxin. Do not mouth pipette and avoid skin contact.

FIBRIN DEGRADATION PRODUCTS

Fibrin is present in the glomerular lesions of several forms of glomerulo-nephritis and fibrin degradation products (FDP) in urine have been considered to be a marker of glomerulonephritis activity and glomerular damage. It was suggested that urinary FDP were the result of fibrinolysis of fibrin within glomerular vessels but it is possible that they arise, like many other urinary proteins, from the filtration of plasma as part of a nonselective proteinuria. While reflecting a degree of glomerular damage, FDP do not necessarily reflect the quantity of fibrin present in the glomerular lesions.

FDP can be measured by inhibition of the agglutination of fibrin-coated tanned erythrocytes by antibody, or by a latex agglutination test which is described below.

Latex test

Kitsets are commercially available (Wellcome Thrombo-Wellco Test) where the latex reagent has been coated with specific antibody against D and E, late fibrinogen-fibrin degradation products (Garvey & Black, 1972). This is a semi-quantitative test which is easy to perform.

The latex suspension is adjusted to give macroscopic agglutination at a concentration of 2 mg/l. Samples giving a positive reaction can then be quantified by diluting the specimen and finding the maximum dilution which produces agglutination.

Any fibrinolytic activity in the specimen is first inhibited and fibrinogen present converted to fibrin by the addition of thrombin before FDP are detected by the sensitized latex particles.

Equipment

Pasteur pipettes—Test tubes 12 × 75 mm—Microscope slides—Orange sticks—Water bath at 37°C—Deep freeze − 30°C—Centrifuge.

Reagents

Latex reagent coated with anti D and E products—Glycine saline buffer pH 8.2—Trasylol (5000 u/ml)—Thrombin—Positive and negative control samples.

Method

(*i*) Add 2 ml urine, preferably at the time of collection to a tube containing 0.1 ml Trasylol to inhibit proteolytic activity.

(*ii*) Shake and then add one drop of concentrated thrombin.

(*iii*) Mix well and freeze quickly at − 30°C. The specimen may be left frozen until the test is due to be performed.

(*iv*) Thaw at 37°C and centrifuge to deposit any particulate matter.

(*v*) Place one drop of supernatant on a slide.

(*vi*) Shake the latex reagent to mix thoroughly, add one drop to the drop of urine already on the slide and mix with an orange stick. Rock the slide gently for up to 2 min and inspect for macroscopic agglutination.

Negative result. Solution remains milky. Report less than 2 mg/l FDP present.

Positive result. Floccular pattern of white particles and clear solution indicates FDP present at 2 mg/l or greater. Prepare dilutions in glycine buffer (pH 8.2) to establish the final dilution giving agglutination.

Controls. Positive and negative control samples should be included with each test.

Normal range. The normal value is less than 0.25 mg/l and the sensitivity of the latex test at 2 mg/l is well above this level. Values between 0.25 mg/l and 2 mg/l could be detected by concentrating the urine by dialysis but the sig-

nificance of levels within this range does not make it worthwhile. Values from
10–100 mg/l are highly significant.

Interpretation
Urine FDP are high in lupus nephritis and proliferative glomerulonephritis,
but only moderately elevated in membranous glomerulonephritis and minimal
change disease. In renal transplantation FDP in urine may be estimated daily;
a rise may indicate the onset of rejection. Overall, FDP in the urine are a general
marker of disease activity but do not correlate well on a daily basis with the
clinical state of the patient.

COMPLEMENT COMPONENTS

The third component C3 has been studied in urine in a range of renal disorders
by several investigators. C3 is not found in the urine of patients with minimal
change disease but is sometimes found in patients suffering from immune
complex-mediated glomerulonephritis. As the urinary excretion does not correlate with the total protein excretion or with selective or nonselective proteinuria
it has been suggested that C3 is derived from complement fixing immune complexes in the glomerulus (Cumming et al, 1976). It is found where the glomerulopathy is progressive and is most common in the urine of patients with membranous glomerulonephritis, mesangiocapillary glomerulonephritis, rapidly
progressive glomerulonephritis and amyloidosis.

Detection of C3
Urine is dialysed against running tap water for eight hours then concentrated
in a solution of polyethylene glycol (Carbowax). C3 is measured by radial immunodiffusion. *See* Single Radial Immunodiffusion in Chapter 2.

BASEMENT MEMBRANE ANTIGENS

The glomerular basement membranes consist of collagenous and noncol-
lagenous glycoprotein components. Glycoproteins with antigenicity similar to
basement membrane have been detected in serum and urine of normal
individuals (McPhaul & Dixon, 1969) as well as in those with renal disease.

Although it is difficult to distinguish glomerular basement membrane from
basement membranes of other organs by their antigens it appears that glycoprotein in the urine of patients with renal disease is derived from damaged
glomerular basement membrane rather than being part of a nonselective
proteinuria.

Glomerular basement membrane (GBM) antigens are detected by radial immunodiffusion using a rabbit antiGBM antiserum. The method is not a routine
test but it does appear that the quantification of GBM antigens in urine may be
used as a measure of glomerular basement membrane damage.

Patients with steroid responsive morphological changes show lower excretion
levels than patients who have more extensive glomerular damage and do not

respond to steroids (Huttenen et al, 1976). Notable quantities are found in the urine of patients with membranous nephritis and lupus nephritis.

ANTIBODY-COATED BACTERIA

The presence of bacteria in the urine is not always an indication of a urinary infection. Attempts to assess the significance of bacteria in urine have led to the introduction of special collection techniques such as suprapubic bladder puncture, particularly in children, and to studies of organisms which are already coated by antibody. It has been suggested that antibody-coated bacteria in the urine are more likely to be found in pyelonephritis than in cystitis and may assist the clinician to determine the site of urinary infection.

Detection of antibody-coated bacteria

Equipment
Conical centrifuge tubes—Test tubes 12 × 75 mm—Microscope slides—Coverslips—Graduated pipettes: 1 ml; 2 ml—Pasteur pipettes—Centrifuge—Fluorescence microscope.

Reagents
FITC polyvalent anti-human-immunoglobulin serum—Phosphate-buffered saline, 0.1M phosphate pH 7.1—Fingernail varnish—Buffered glycerol mountant.

Method
A urine sample, preferably obtained by suprapubic aspiration of the bladder, is delivered to the laboratory as soon as possible.

(*i*) Centrifuge the sample and wash the deposit twice in the phosphate-buffered saline, which contains 15 mM sodium azide to suppress growth of microorganisms. Resuspend the sediment in 2 ml PBS.

(*ii*) To a glass test tube, add 0.2 ml washed urine sediment and 0.05 ml FITC polyvalent anti-human immunoglobulin serum and incubate for 30 min at 37°C.

(*iii*) Centrifuge and wash twice in 2 ml PBS.

(*iv*) Prepare a smear from the washed deposit on a clean glass microscope slide and dry in air.

(*v*) Mount under coverslip using buffered glycerol. Seal preparation with nail varnish.

(*vi*) Examine the preparation on the fluorescence microscope, both by ultraviolet and narrow-band blue illumination (Nairn, 1976). Using a × 100 objective, count all bacteria noting those showing specific immunofluorescent staining in each field, until at least 20 bacteria have been counted. A positive test is one which shows at least 20% of organisms coated with immunoglobulin. Total organism counting is best done by darkground transmitted tungsten light, with incident mercury lamp illumination for fluorescent organisms.

Controls. (*i*) Normal rabbit serum conjugated with FITC should give no fluorescent staining. (*ii*) Pretreatment with 0.05 ml unconjugated polyvalent antiserum added to 0.2 ml of the washed test specimen, incubated for 30 min at 37°C, washed twice and then tested with specific FITC-labelled antiglobulin as above, (the blocking test) should inhibit staining. (*iii*) After microbiological isolation of the organism from the urine, a suspension prepared from a sub-culture in 0.2 ml PBS is stained with the FITC-polyvalent anti–human immunoglobulin serum to assess non-specific binding of the conjugated antiserum. Such a bacterial preparation might be stainable by indirect immunofluorescence with the patient's own serum as first layer; this could establish the presence of specific antibacterial serum antibody.

Significance
Antibody which covers bacteria may not be directed specifically against the micro-organism but may have been absorbed non-specifically from immuno-globulins present in the urine.

Gram-positive organisms appear to bind immunoglobulins in the urine in a non-specific manner and their presence does not indicate a particular site of infection.

Yeasts coated with antibody, often strongly, do not indicate whether kidney or bladder are principally involved.

On the other hand, Gram-negative organisms coated with antibody are most frequently found in acute pyelonephritis. The percentage of positive tests is highest in adults, ranging from 60–100%, and is reduced to a level of 30–40% in infants and children. The lower incidence in children may result from their presentation earlier in the course of the illness before an antibody response has been fully developed.

Tests may also be carried out using monospecific antisera against IgG, IgA and IgM. Antibodies coating bacteria usually include the IgG class although IgM may also be present.

It is not yet clear that the detection of antibody-coated gram-negative bacteria is helpful in distinguishing upper from lower renal tract infection. In children examined by the bladder washout technique, Hellerstein et al (1978) detected antibody-coated bacteria in 66% of patients with upper urinary tract infection and 40% of patients with lower urinary tract infection and expressed reservations about the usefulness of the technique.

REFERENCES

Cumming A D, Thomson D, Davison A M, Robson J S 1976 Significance of urinary C3 excretion in glomerulonephritis. Journal of Clinical Pathology 29: 601–607
Garvey M B, Black J M 1972 The detection of fibrinogen/fibrin degradation products by means of a new antibody-coated latex particle. Journal of Clinical Pathology 25: 680–682
Hellerstein S, Kennedy E, Nussbaum L, Rice K 1978 Localization of the site of urinary tract infections by means of antibody-coated bacteria in the urinary sediments. The Journal of Pediatrics 92: 188–193
Huttunen N-P, Hallman N, Rapola J 1976 Glomerular basement membrane antigens in congenital and acquired nephrotic syndrome in childhood. Nephron 16: 401–414
McPhaul J J, Dixon F J 1969 Basement membrane antigens in serum and urine. Transplantation Proceedings 1: 964–967
Nairn R C 1976 Fluorescent Protein Tracing. 4th edn. Churchill Livingstone, Edinburgh

UNCITED BIBLIOGRAPHY

Beetham R, Mills R J, Raine D N, White R H R 1974 Some analytical aspects of the immunochemical determination of the selectivity of proteinuria. Annals of Clinical Biochemistry 11: 59–66

Bienenstock J, Poortmans J 1970 Renal clearance of 15 plasma proteins in renal disease. Journal of Laboratory and Clinical Medicine 75: 297–306

Boesken W H, Kopf K, Schollmeyer P 1973 Differentiation of proteinuric diseases by discelectrophoretic molecular weight analysis of urinary proteins. Clinical Nephrology 1: 311–318

Brenner B M, Hostetter T H, Humes H D 1978 Molecular basis of proteinuria of glomerular origin. New England Journal of Medicine 298: 826–833

Bretscher M S 1971 Major human erythrocyte glycoprotein spans the cell membrane. Nature New Biology 231: 229–232

Cachera C, Mizon C, Fruchart J-C, Mizon J, Tacquet A 1978 Application de l'electrophorese en gel de polyacrylamide—SDS a l'etude des proteinuries. Annales de Biologie Clinique 36: 27–32

Hardwicke J 1975 Laboratory aspects of proteinuria in human disease. Clinical Nephrology 3: 37–41

Hobbs J R 1975 Bence-Jones Proteins. Essays in Medical Biochemistry ed Marks V, Hales C N 1: 105–131 Biochemical Society, London

Lizana J, Brito M, Davis M R 1977 Assessment of five quantitative methods for determination of total proteins in urine. Clinical Biochemistry 10: 89–93

Manuel Y, Revillard J P, Betuel H (ed) 1970 Proteins in Normal and Pathological Urine. Karger, Basel

Pesce A J 1974 Methods used for the analysis of proteins in the urine. Nephron 13: 93–104

Pesce A J, Gaizutis M, Pollak V E 1970 Selectivity of proteinuria: An evaluation of the immunochemical and gel filtration techniques. Journal of Laboratory and Clinical Medicine 75: 586–606

Pesce A J, Hsu A, Kornhauser C, Sethi K, Ooi B S, Pollak V E 1976 Method for measuring the concentration of urinary proteins according to their molecular size category. Clinical Chemistry 22: 667–672

Pollak V E (ed) 1974 Symposium on Proteinuria. Nephron 13: 1–104

Savory J, Pu P H, Sunderman F W 1968 A biuret method for determination of protein in normal urine. Clinical Chemistry 14: 1160–1171

Weber K, Pringle J. R, Osborn M 1972 Measurement of molecular weights by electrophoresis on SDS acrylamide gel. In: Methods of Enzymology ed Hirs C H W, Timasheff S N vol 26 p 3–27 Academic Press, New York and London

7
The Renal Biopsy

A. R. McGiven

SPECIMEN PREPARATION

The typical renal biopsy specimen is a cylindrical core of tissue measuring 1–2 cm in length and 2–3 mm in diameter. It is customary, using a new razor blade for each biopsy, to slice 2 mm off each end for electron microscopic examination and to bisect the remainder longitudinally so that one half may be examined by conventional histology and the other half by immunofluorescence. Occasionally the biopsy will be fragmented and an arbitrary selection must be made. Some workers advocate examining the specimen under the dissecting microscope to identify renal cortex before dividing the material. Each fragment should be placed in its appropriate fixative. For histological examination the specimen is fixed in Helly's fluid then processed and serial sections stained with H and E, PAS, and methenamine silver stains. For electron microscopy the specimen is fixed in osmium tetroxide. Increasing use is being made of thin plastic-embedded sections for light microscopy. Material for immuno-fluorescence may be placed in saline for transport to the laboratory.

Examination by immunofluorescence
A full account of general procedures is given by Nairn (1976).

Equipment and reagents
See Antinuclear antibodies.—Immunofluorescence in Chapter 5.

Freezing of samples
Before sectioning for immunofluorescence studies the specimen must be frozen. Ideally this is done rapidly to prevent distortion of the tissue by ice crystal formation. Several methods are available.

Basically the specimen is embedded horizontally in a mound of Tissue Tek Compound OCT freezing medium on a small piece of cork, or within an aluminium foil float or mould. The specimen is then handled with forceps by the cork or foil and plunged into the freezing mixture which may be isopentane cooled previously in liquid nitrogen or a liquid nitrogen-isopentane slurry (Nairn, 1976). The cork may then be attached to the chuck pre-cooled below −20°C by a small amount of OCT or the foil stripped off and the block of OCT frozen to the chuck by a few drops of water. If a dry ice-ethanol mixture is used for freezing care must be taken not to let the tissue come into contact with the mixture as this may harden the specimen and make sectioning difficult. If the above methods are not possible adequate sections can still be obtained from specimens frozen in OCT on the chuck in the cryostat. The specimen is then cut in the cryostat or stored on the chuck at $-20°C$ or below in a closed container. If it is not possible to snap-freeze the specimen shortly after the biopsy has been taken, it may be left in physiological saline at $4°C$ overnight.

Sections

Section cutting is one of the most important steps in the processing of the renal biopsy. The aim is to produce thin sections of even thickness which are not curled up and remain on the slide during the various washing and staining steps. Cryostats assist by maintaining the cold temperature of the knife blade and provide a guide plate on which flat sections rest, from which they can be retrieved directly on to chemically clean glass slides. The position of the specimen in the OCT block, orientation on the chuck, the angle of the knife blade and the skill and experience of the section cutter are important factors which influence the quality of the sections. Sections $4\,\mu m$ in thickness are cut on a cryostat at $-20°C$ and air-dried by a fan for 3 h at room temperature or at $4°C$ overnight. Adequate drying is important so that the section will remain adherent to the slide and not become detached during staining and washing.

Initially 48 sections are cut and mounted in pairs on 24 slides numbered consecutively. It is helpful to place two sections a few mm apart on each slide and to indicate their position by drawing a circle on the undersurface of the slide with a marker which identifies the area for staining, mounting the coverslip and examination. The provision of duplicate sections does not significantly reduce the selection of material available for separate staining procedures and apart from being helpful in the event of one section becoming folded or washed off provides a wider selection of material for examination and photography. The brightness of immunofluorescent staining is inevitably reduced by exposures for photography and the extra section allows demonstration of the original brilliance to interested clinicians or laboratory staff at the conclusion of the examination.

Suitability of sections for immunofluorescence examination. This must be considered in the context of the patient's disorder as the physician may wish to repeat the biopsy immediately if the specimen is unsatisfactory. Slides 1, 12 and 24 are stained by Paragon and examined by light microscopy to determine if the specimen is suitable for immunofluorescence examination. First observe if kidney tissue is present and note the number of glomeruli; sometimes the tissue proves to be portions of muscle, liver or fat. If no glomeruli are present in the first set of 24 slides, then a further 12 and if possible 24 should be prepared and numbers 36 and 48 examined. The presence and number of glomeruli is a guide to suitability of preparations for immunofluorescence examination. Commonly one stains sections from slide 2 onwards, from slide 23 backwards, or sections on either side of slide 12.

If glomeruli are not present in the first 24 slides it is sometimes possible to find them in deeper sections, and there is a responsibility to the patient to screen all of the specimen under these circumstances. If glomeruli are absent useful information can still be obtained about tubules, vessels and interstitium to warrant processing the specimen. Even if glomeruli do not appear to be present on screening by light microscopy, immunofluorescence staining may highlight unsuspected glomeruli or portions of glomeruli in the section. A portion of a glomerulus may be sufficient to confirm a clinical diagnosis of IgA nephropathy, Goodpasture's syndrome, membranous glomerulonephritis or other immune-complex disorder. Thus there are good reasons for staining sections regardless of whether or not glomeruli appear to be present.

Fluorescein-conjugated antisera
The following antisera labelled with fluorescein isothiocyanate (FITC) form a battery of useful reagents:
   Routine — (*i*) Polyvalent antiglobulin — (*ii*) Anti-IgG — (*iii*) Anti-IgM — (*iv*) Anti-IgA — (*v*) Anti-albumin — (*vi*) Anti-fibrin — (*viii*) Anti-Clq — (*viii*) Anti-C3 — (*ix*) Anti-C4 — (*x*) Anti-properdin.
   As required — (*i*) Anti-Hepatitis B antigen — (*ii*) Anti-kappa light chain — (*iii*) Anti-lambda light chain.
   All of the above FITC antisera are available commercially. Most can be used at a dilution of 1 : 10 in phosphate-buffered saline 0.1M pH 7.1 (PBS). This reduces non-specific immunofluorescence as well as allowing economical use of the reagent. Antisera differ in their potency and the optimum dilution should be determined for each reagent. Diluted sera should be stored frozen in appropriate aliquots (0.5 or 1.0 ml) to reduce the number of occasions a sample is thawed and refrozen.
   For various reasons some laboratories may wish to use an even wider range of antisera. A number of reports list the detection of properdin as a marker of alternative pathway activation of complement but satisfactory sera may be difficult to acquire.

Staining procedures
Non-specific background staining may result from a film of plasma proteins formed over sections during preparation and also from proteins trapped in glomeruli. Indeed glomeruli in some normal individuals may give a linear staining pattern and mimic that seen in Goodpasture's syndrome. Before staining, it is helpful to wash sections to reduce background effects and to remove OCT medium from around the tissue on the slide. Sections which have been dried in air by a fan at room temperature for 3 h or at 4°C overnight are first washed for 15 min in PBS, allowed to dry at room temperature and then covered with one drop of commercial antiserum which has been diluted 1 in 10 with PBS. The sections are left in a moist atmosphere for 30 min, washed twice for at least 5 min in PBS and then mounted in buffered glycerol-saline. We recommend equal Parts of A.R. glycerol and isotonic veronal-buffered saline—10.3 g sodium veronal, 6.2 g NaCl, HCl to pH 8.6, to 1 litre with distilled water (Nairn, 1976).

Fluorescence microscopy
Specimens may be examined by darkground ultraviolet and narrow-band blue

illumination with a wide angle condenser or by incident light illumination. Mercury vapour lamps (HB200) provide strong excitation which is further enhanced by modern optical filter systems designed for FITC (Nairn, 1976).

Photographs of individual lesions are recorded on colour or black and white film. Colour slides are most useful to demonstrate findings later. Excellent black and white photographs can be made from the monochrome green images obtained by narrow-band blue illumination, either directly or via colour transparencies. With such illumination, close to the absorption maximum of FITC (495 nm), background autofluorescence is much less than with ultraviolet excitation. The latter, with a colourless barrier filter reveals general tissue architecture better and provides attractive, polychromatic colour transparencies with green FITC fluorescence against a blue autofluorescent background.

IMMUNOFLUORESCENCE MORPHOLOGY

Examination of the specimen should be carried out systematically and preferably after having studied the appearances of the Paragon-stained sections. It is important to observe the distribution and intensity of fluorescent staining and note any characteristic patterns in glomeruli, tubules, vessels and interstitium.

Glomerular immunofluorescence patterns

Staining may occur in the capillary loops, mesangium, Bowman's capsule and Bowman's space.

Capillary loops
Granular. Soluble immune complexes formed in antigen excess in the circulation are trapped in the capillary wall to give a pattern variously referred to as

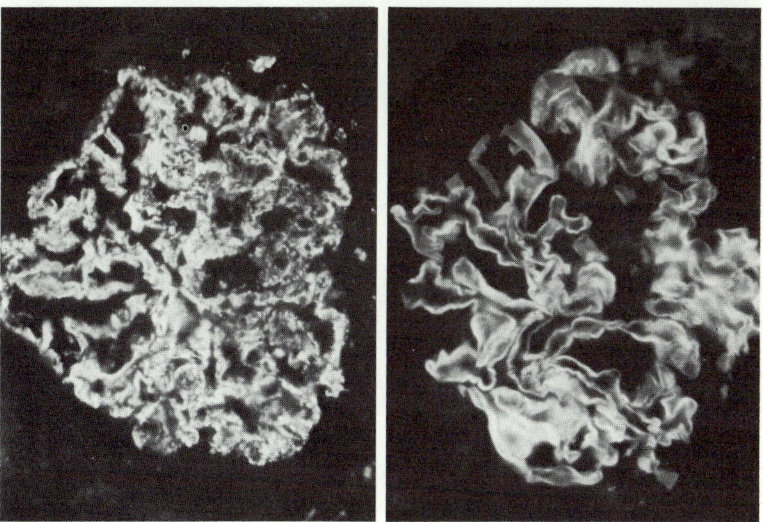

Figure 7.1. Glomerulus shows diffuse fine speckled staining of IgG in capillary loops. This pattern indicates immune-complex nephropathy.
Figure 7.2. Glomerulus shows linear basement membrane staining for IgG. This pattern indicates localization of antiglomerular basement membrane antibody.

granular, lumpy, stippled or speckled (Fig. 7.1). Precise localization of deposits in a subepithelial, intramembranous or subendothelial position usually requires confirmation from electron microscopy or the examination of 1 μm plastic-embedded sections. As deposits enlarge they may overlap in the section and appear confluent, giving an appearance which may require close examination to distinguish it from a linear antiglomerular basement membrane staining pattern.

Linear. Deposition of antiglomerular basement membrane antibody results in sharp delineation of the basement membrane by immunoglobulins (Fig. 7.2). Associated complement deposition is usually segmental with intervening unstained areas. Linear staining from the trapping of globulin is seen in some normal kidneys and in diabetes mellitus and may occasionally cause difficulties in renal biopsy interpretation, which can usually be resolved by referring to the clinical history.

Mesangium

Circulating immune complexes of the intermediate type, larger than those that deposit in the periphery of loops (*i.e.* $> 10^6$ daltons), may be deposited in the mesangium.

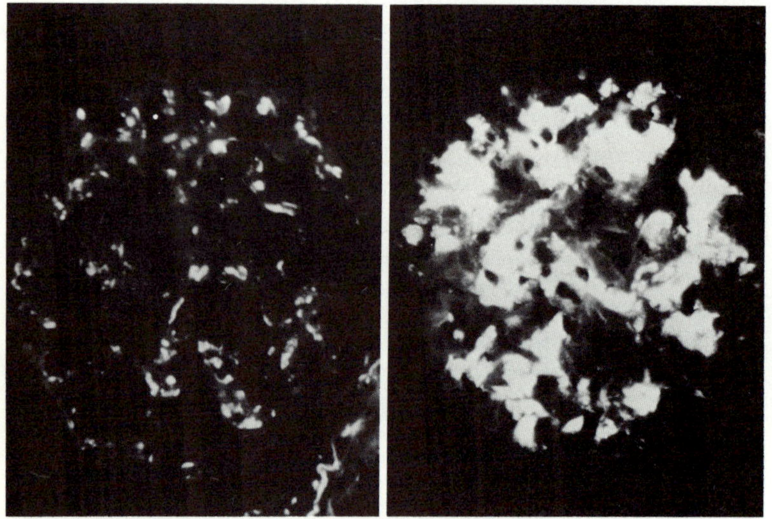

Figure 7.3. Glomerulus shows comma shaped deposits of IgA. This pattern indicates early mesangiopathic nephropathy.

Figure 7.4. Glomerulus shows prominent mesangial deposits of IgG. Advanced mesangiopathic process, in this instance in a patient with systemic lupus erythematosus.

Comma. The earliest mesangial deposits often occur at the base of a loop and abut on the adjacent subendothelial region in the loop (Fig. 7.3).

Branching. Deposits expand the mesangium in mesangiopathic forms of glomerulonephritis giving first a branching axial pattern and later a lobulated or clover leaf pattern (Fig. 7.4).

Aggregates. Focal deposits of variable size and irregular shape occur in a random fashion and may accompany other patterns of immune complex deposition (Fig. 7.5).

Bowman's capsule
Linear or scattered aggregates are seen sometimes in the parietal layer of Bowman's capsule.

Bowman's space
Plasma proteins may be found within Bowman's space. It is unusual to detect albumin here even in patients with nephrotic syndrome as albumin is retained poorly in the sections unless it is within cells. Fibrin may be found, particularly

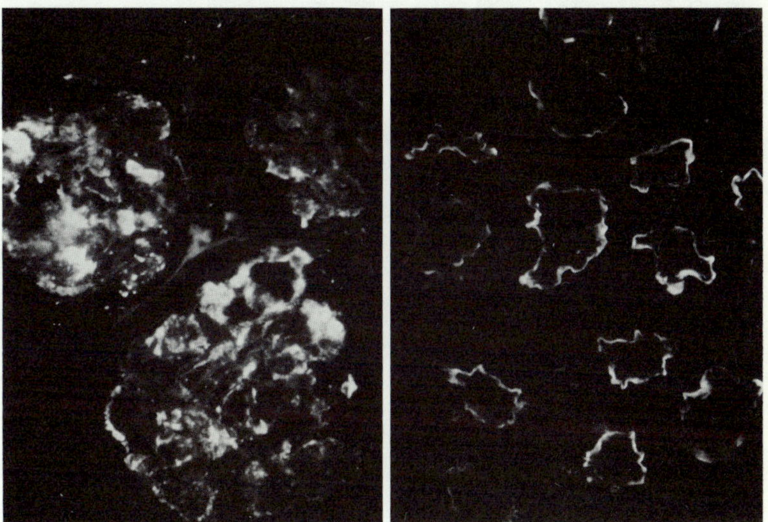

Figure 7.5. Glomeruli show mesangial aggregates of IgM together with speckled deposits. Mixed mesangial and loop pattern.
Figure 7.6. Tubules show linear basement membrane staining for IgG. This pattern indicates antitubular basement membrane antibody deposition.

if associated with crescents. Recently Tamm-Horsfall protein has been detected here (McGiven et al, 1978)—possibly a sign of intratubular reflux as this glycoprotein which is a prominent component of tubular casts is produced by cells of the ascending limb of the loop of Henle and distal tubule.

Tubular immunofluorescence patterns

Basement membrane
Linear. In this pattern there is continuous linear staining of the basement membrane of tubules and it appears to be due to the localization of antibodies and complement reacting with tubular basement membrane (Fig. 7.6). Usually the staining is uneven with some tubules staining strongly and others not at all. Albumin and $\alpha 1$ anti-trypsin are commonly found in this region.

Segmental. Short sections of tubular basement membrane show a linear pattern.

Granular. Irregular patchy deposits are present in the tubular basement membrane region (Fig. 7.7).

Cytoplasm
Protein droplets, predominantly albumin but sometimes other plasma proteins may be found in clusters within the cytoplasm of tubular cells and in most

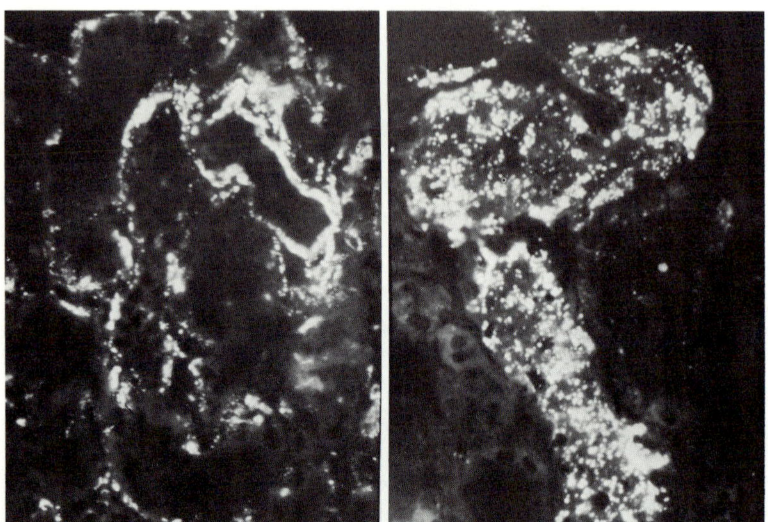

Figure 7.7. Prominent speckled deposits of C1q in tubular basement membrane region. This pattern suggests tubular immune deposits in a patient with systemic lupus erythematosus.
Figure 7.8. Prominent albumin droplets in tubular cytoplasm. This pattern is seen in many forms of glomerulonephritis.

cases probably indicate tubular reabsorption of protein (Fig. 7.8). Secretory IgA is normally present in tubular cytoplasm.

Casts
Casts within the lumen of tubules commonly stain for a variety of plasma proteins and not only albumin. Complement components, particularly C3 usually accompany immunoglobulins and Tamm-Horsfall protein. IgA may be particularly conspicuous.

Vascular immunofluorescence patterns
Arterioles and interlobular arteries frequently show plasma proteins within their walls (Fig. 7.9). These may give homogeneous or segmental patterns. The most frequently identified component is C3 but immunoglobulins and fibrin are not uncommonly found. Sometimes staining may only involve the lumen, as in fibrin deposition associated with thrombus formation. No distinction is made in this chapter between fibrinogen and fibrin as routine FITC antisera react with each.

Interstitial immunofluorescence patterns
No specific patterns are found and most obvious staining is probably due to leakage of the contents of damaged tubules or vessels either due to disease or

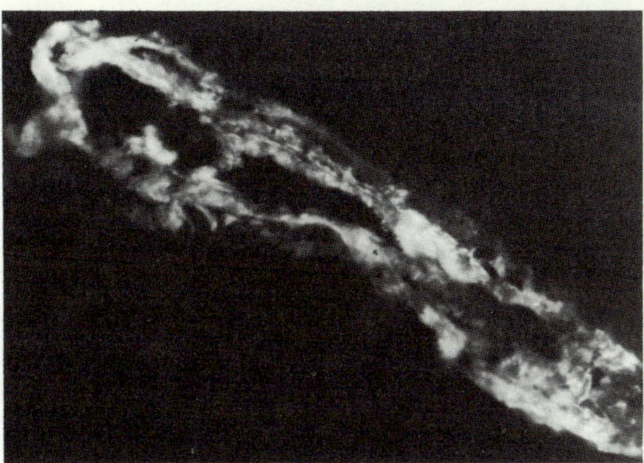

Figure 7.9. Interlobular artery shows intramural staining for C1q.

during processing. Small deposits in peritubular vessels may give staining which is difficult to distinguish from tubular staining. Plasma proteins, particularly fibrin, may be conspicuous in the lumen of peritubular vessels and is seen in normal biopsy material.

INTERPRETATION OF IMMUNOFLUORESCENCE APPEARANCES

Several of the above patterns indicate a particular type of immunopathological process but are not in themselves diagnostic for a single disease entity. Many occur in combination and a precise clinical and pathological diagnosis is usually only arrived at after consideration of the histological appearances supplemented by electron microscopy and consultation with the patient's physician.

Glomeruli

(*i*) *Diffuse granular pattern involving capillary loops.* This pattern is commonly seen in acute diffuse proliferative (post-streptococcal) glomerulonephritis and membranous nephritis and can also be seen in mesangiocapillary glomerulo-nephritis and systemic lupus erythematosus.

(*ii*) *Granular deposits involving loops with irregular aggregates in mesangium.* This pattern occurs in systemic lupus erythematosus and other immune com-plex nephropathies, often of undetermined origin.

(*iii*) *Focal glomerular aggregates, mainly mesangial without obvious loop involvement.* Focal sclerosing glomerulonephritis may show irregular deposits predominantly of IgM with C3.

(*iv*) *Comma-shaped deposits in axial region.* These are frequently seen and represent mesangial localization of immune deposits. It is an early finding in IgA nephropathy and Henoch-Schönlein syndrome but is seen in other immune complex nephropathies.

(*v*) *Mesangial aggregates often communicating in axial region to give branching pattern*. This pattern is characteristic of IgA nephropathy, where IgA deposition may be associated with IgG and C3. Henoch Schönlein syndrome gives a similar picture. It may also occur in systemic lupus erythematosus.

(*vi*) *Segmental staining of capillary loops*. Short segments of capillary loops may stain with reagents to give a segmental linear staining pattern. In many cases this can be seen to be due to confluence of small deposits but in other cases it may represent a prominent subendothelial deposit as in systemic lupus erythematosus.

(*vii*) *Linear staining of capillary loops*. Patients with Goodpasture's syndrome show linear basement membrane staining due to IgG deposition. Associated C3 deposition is not usually linear and shows a patchy staining pattern.

Vessels

Plasma proteins are sometimes found in walls of interlobular arteries and afferent arterioles and in some instances the deposition is continuous with an affected area in the glomerulus. C3 is the component usually detected but immunoglobulins and fibrin may also be seen on occasions. C3 in vessels is frequently found as an isolated immunofluorescence finding in the absence of significant morphological changes, an observation that is unexplained.

About one quarter of patients with IgA nephropathy also show IgA in afferent arterioles.

Fibrin is expected as part of the vasculosis in hypertension but is not found as often as one might anticipate.

Tubules

Granular and irregular deposits related to tubular basement membrane may be seen in systemic lupus erythematosus. Linear staining by immunoglobulins and complement is frequently found in transplanted kidneys showing evidence of rejection, and is also found in some patients with interstitial nephritis particularly in patients who have received methicillin.

Interstitium

Aggregates of immunoglobulins and complement have been reported in systemic lupus erythematosus. Proteinaceous material may be of obvious significance in interstitial nephritis, and Tamm-Horsfall protein presumably released from damaged tubules has been implicated as a possible cause of an autoimmune interstitial nephritis.

Nature of plasma protein deposits

The composition of plasma protein aggregates may change during the development and resolution of an immunologically mediated process in the same fashion that appearances may change on light microscopy during the course of a disease. Initial immunological damage is associated with immunoglobulin and complement deposition, but as the disease progresses albumin and fibrin may accumulate when exudation follows vascular damage. Usually IgG is the predominant immunoglobulin and C3 the predominant complement component. However, traces at least of IgA and IgM are common in immune complex nephropathies, and in lupus nephritis IgA, IgG and IgM are frequently conspicuous. IgM aggregates are common in focal glomerulosclerosis. Although IgD and IgE have been reported in glomeruli, no consistent pattern has emerged and the use of antisera against these immunoglobulins in the routine examination of renal biopsies is not yet justified.

C1q is frequently seen in immune complex nephropathies and may become less prominent as the disease continues. When present, C4 tends to mirror C3 but usually gives weaker staining. The presence of C1q and/or C4 indicates activation of the conventional complement pathway but does not exclude associated alternative pathway activity. The presence of properdin is assumed to indicate alternative pathway activation.

C3 may be found in a speckled patchy pattern in the absence of immunoglobulin deposition. This has been noted in some patients with hypocomplementaemic mesangiocapillary glomerulonephritis. There are theoretical explanations why C3 may be detected in the absence of immunoglobulins, such as the masking of antibody by antigen, but the question is unresolved. In some cases it may not indicate an immunological event. To decide if C3 deposition is immunologically determined, Lachman & Hobart (1978) recommend washing sections in 2 M NaCl before staining. Exuded protein will be eluted but strongly membrane bound complement components will remain.

WHAT PROBLEMS CAN RENAL BIOPSY IMMUNOFLUORESCENCE SOLVE?

(*i*) It can determine whether the kidney shows evidence of immunologically mediated disease, when light microscopy appearances are within normal limits or show only minor changes as in IgA nephropathy and early membranous or lupus nephritis.

(*ii*) It permits a firm diagnosis of Goodpasture's syndrome, provided the linear basement membrane staining found in some normal kidneys is not misinterpreted. Usually patients with Goodpasture's syndrome have staining of greater intensity than that found sometimes in normal kidneys; the clinical history as well as serological tests for glomerular basement membrane antibodies will help resolve the occasional doubtful case.

(*iii*) It provides a firm diagnosis of IgA nephropathy and confirms Henoch Schönlein syndrome by IgA deposition mainly in mesangium.

(*iv*) It confirms immune complex disease in proliferative glomerulonephritis, membranous glomerulonephritis and mesangiocapillary glomerulonephritis.

(*v*) It confirms or refutes a diagnosis of lupus nephritis when antinuclear antibodies of doubtful significance are present.

(*vi*) It may distinguish focal glomerulosclerosis from focal sclerosis following immune complex nephropathy by revealing granular staining in residual capillary loops in the latter.

(*vii*) Negative immunofluorescence may confirm a diagnosis of minimal change disease (lipoid nephrosis).

(*viii*) Tubular basement membrane staining in a transplanted kidney indicates antirenal activity.

Table 7.1. Diagnostic factors in glomerulonephritis

Disease	Kidney		Serum				Urine	Other
	Histology	Immunofluore-scence	Proteins	Complement	Immune complexes	Streptococcal antibodies		
Minimal change	Normal	Negative or traces Ig	↓Albumin	N	50%	N	Selective proteinuria	EM fused foot processes, nephrotic syndrome
Diffuse proliferative glomerulonephritis	Diffuse proliferative	Granular IgG, IgA, IgM, C1q, C4, C3, properdin	↑Globulin	↓C3, ↓C4	80%	↑	Nonselective proteinuria, RBC, casts, FDP	EM deposits in loops and mesangium, extramembranous humps, C3 splitting factors
Mesangioproliferative glomerulonephritis	Segmental proliferative	Variable IgM, C3, C4	N	N	20%	N	Selective proteinuria, RBC	EM mesangial deposits, nephrotic syndrome
Mesangiocapillary glomerulonephritis	Membrano-proliferative	Granular C3 ± Ig	↓Albumin	↓C3	50%	N	Nonselective proteinuria, RBC	EM subendothelial deposits, C3NeF, nephrotic syndrome
Dense deposit disease	Membrano-proliferative	Patchy C3 or negative	↓Albumin	↓C3	50%	N	Proteinuria, RBC	EM dense thickened glomerular basement membrane, Bowman's capsule and tubules affected sometimes, C3NeF, nephrotic syndrome
Membranous glomerulonephritis	Basement membrane thickening	Granular IgG, IgA, IgM, C1q, C3, C4	↓Albumin	N	30%	N	Nonselective proteinuria, RBC	EM deposits in basement membrane and mesangium, nephrotic syndrome
Focal glomerulosclerosis	Segmental sclerosis	Aggregates IgM, C3, C4	↓Albumin	N or ↓	50%	N	Nonselective proteinuria, RBC	Nephrotic syndrome, responds poorly to corticosteroids
Goodpasture's syndrome	Proliferative with crescents	Linear IgG, C3, fibrin	N	N	25%	N	Proteinuria, RBC	Lung haemorrhage, serum antiGBM antibodies
Rapidly progressive glomerulonephritis	Proliferative with crescents	Granular IgG, IgM, C3, fibrin	N	↓C3	N or ↑	N or ↑	Proteinuria, RBC	Sometimes poststreptococcal
IgA nephropathy	Mesangioproliferative	Mesangial IgA, IgG, C3, properdin, fibrin	↑IgA	N	30%	N	Proteinuria, RBC	Recurrent haematuria, may follow respiratory infections

Table 7.2. Diagnostic factors of renal disease in systemic disorders

Disease	Kidney		Serum				Urine	Other
	Histology	Immunofluore-scence	Proteins	Complement	Immune complexes	Streptococcal antibodies		
Systemic lupus erythematosus	Minimal, membranous, focal proliferative, diffuse proliferative	Granular IgG, IgA, IgM, C1q, C3, C4, C3PA, properdin	Globulin	$\downarrow$C3, $\downarrow$C4	50–80%	N	Proteinuria, FDP	EM subendothelial deposits, ANA, skin band test
Scleroderma	Mucoid intimal thickening, focal necrosis	Sometimes IgG C3, fibrin	N or $\uparrow$Globulin	N	N	N	Proteinuria	Speckled ANA, rheumatoid factor, antinucleolar antibody, skin manifestations
Henoch-Schönlein syndrome	Mesangioproliferative, crescents	Mesangial IgA, IgG, C3, properdin, fibrin	$\uparrow$IgA	N	30%	N	Proteinuria, RBC	Rash, abdominal pain, arthritis
Amyloidosis	Amyloid deposits in glomeruli and vessels	Usually negative	$\downarrow$Albumin, $\uparrow$Globulin	N	N	N	Nonselective proteinuria	EM fibrils 800 nm diameter, beading 500 nm
Multiple myeloma	Interstitial nephritis	Casts stain for protein	$\uparrow$Globulin, M protein	N	N	N	Bence-Jones proteinuria	Paraproteinaemia
Polyarteritis nodosa	Vasculitis, focal necrosis, crescents	Fibrin	N or $\uparrow$Globulin	N or $\downarrow$	30 − 70%	N	Proteinuria, FDP, RBC	Associated with drugs, hepatitis B antigenaemia, systemic vasculitis
Wegener's granulomatosis	Focal proliferation, necrosis	Variable fibrin, Ig, C3	$\uparrow$IgA, $\uparrow$IgG, $\downarrow$IgM	N or $\uparrow$	20%	N	Proteinuria, RBC, casts, WBC	Respiratory tract involvement
Haemolytic uraemic syndrome	Thrombi, focal necrosis, crescents	Fibrin	N	N or $\downarrow$C3	N	N	Nonselective proteinuria, RBC, casts, FDP	Thrombocytopenia, commonly in infants
Diabetes mellitus	Diffuse or focal mesangial sclerosis	Nonspecific linear IgG, variable aggregates	N	N	N	N	Proteinuria, glycosuria	Retinal microangiopathy

IMMUNOFLUORESCENCE PATTERNS IN PARTICULAR DISEASES

Diagnostic features of glomerulonephritis and nephropathies associated with systemic disorders are tabulated in Tables 7.1 and 7.2 respectively.

Minimal change (minor glomerular abnormality)

Immunofluorescence staining is usually negative but traces of plasma proteins may be present occasionally in glomeruli. Under these circumstances, when IgM is found, the possibility of focal glomerulosclerosis should be considered.

Histologically the glomeruli are normal or show only mild changes. Tubular cells may be vacuolated and contain protein droplets.

Electron microscopy reveals fusion of epithelial cell foot processes.

This condition is a common cause of the nephrotic syndrome, particularly in children. Although immune complexes have been found in the blood they are not detected in glomeruli and the pathogenesis of the condition is not known. The nephrotic syndrome usually responds to corticosteroid therapy and the prognosis is good.

Diffuse proliferative glomerulonephritis

All glomeruli show a diffuse granular pattern of staining particularly for IgG and C3, but IgM, C1q, C4 and properdin may also be present. Deposits may occur in the mesangium as well as in capillary loops (Fig. 7.10). The pattern is consistent with the deposition of circulating immune complexes and in some cases streptococcal antigens have been demonstrated in the glomeruli.

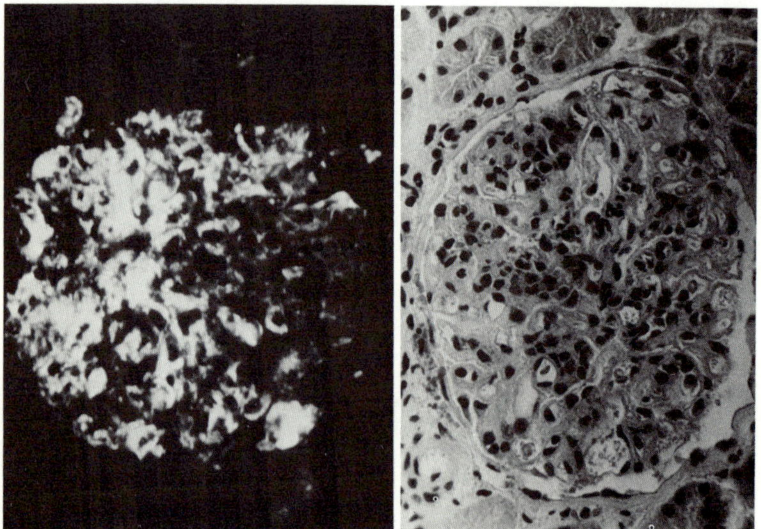

Figure 7.10. Glomerulus shows numerous deposits of C3 in mesangium and capillary loops. Diffuse proliferative glomerulonephritis.

Figure 7.11. Glomerulus is hypercellular and shows some neutrophil infiltration. Diffuse proliferative glomerulonephritis. H & E.

Histologically the glomeruli show a proliferation of endothelial and mesangial cells, often accompanied by neutrophil infiltration (7.11).

Electron microscopy reveals electron-dense deposits, in some cases as humps projecting from the external aspect of the basement membrane of capillary loops (Fig. 7.12).

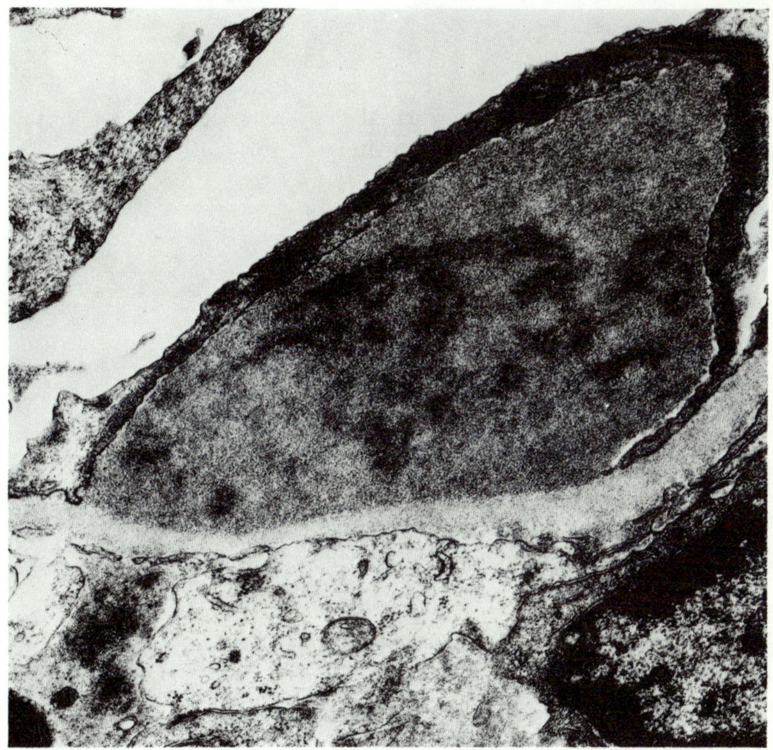

Figure 7.12. Electron micrograph shows electron-dense subepithelial deposit. Diffuse proliferative glomerulonephritis.

Clinically this condition is usually associated with haematuria but some patients have the nephrotic syndrome. Streptococcal antibody tests are likely to be positive and serum C3 levels are usually depressed but return to normal in 8–12 weeks in uncomplicated cases. Serum C3 splitting factors are present in some patients.

Mesangioproliferative glomerulonephritis

Glomeruli showing mesangioproliferative changes which are not associated with IgA nephropathy or systemic lupus erythematosus may have a variable pattern of immunoglobulin and complement deposition, presumably due to the accumulation of immune complexes (Fig. 7.13). IgG, IgM, C3 and fibrin may be found.

Histologically there is a variable increase in mesangial cellularity and expansion of mesangial matrix (7.14).

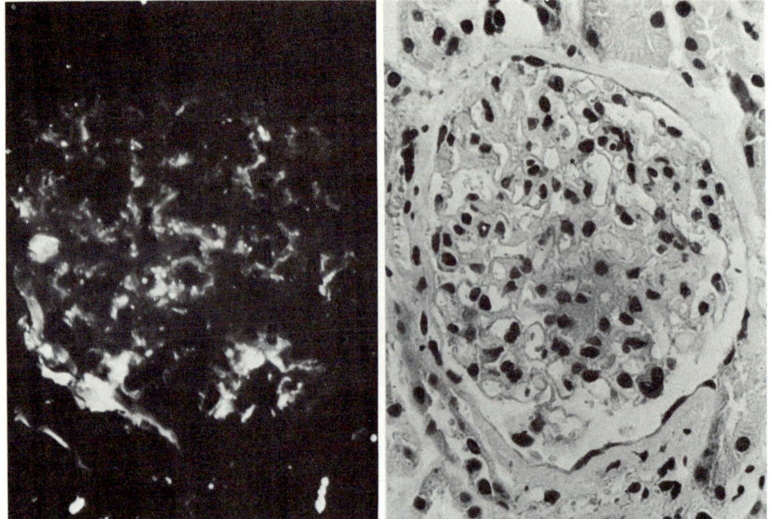

Figure 7.13. Glomerulus shows deposits of C3 most prominent in mesangium.
Mesangioproliferative glomerulonephritis.
Figure 7.14. Glomerulus shows expansion of mesangial matrix. Mesangioproliferative
glomerulonephritis. H & E.

Electron microscopy reveals electron-dense deposits in the mesangium.

Mesangioproliferative glomerulonephritis should be distinguished from
mesangiocapillary glomerulonephritis and resolving acute proliferative
glomerulonephritis.

Mesangiocapillary glomerulonephritis (membranoproliferative glomerulonephritis)

Granular deposits staining for immunoglobulins and complement may be
found in capillary loops, or C3 alone often in a rather peripheral location (Fig.
7.15).

In this form of nephritis there is proliferation of mesangial cells (Fig. 7.16)
which extend into adjacent capillary loops beneath the endothelium. In some
areas there is duplication of the basement membrane to give a double contour
appearance with silver stains (Fig. 7.17).

Electron-dense deposits may be seen, particularly in a subendothelial location.

The nature of the antigen–antibody reaction concerned is not usually known.
Hypocomplementaemia and C3NeF are associated with this condition and there
are indications of complement activation by both classical and alternative pathways.

Dense deposit disease

Although appearances are variable, circumscribed aggregates of C3 may be
present in glomeruli (Fig. 7.18).

This condition is also referred to as mesangiocapillary glomerulonephritis
Type II, and histologically is one of the membranoproliferative forms of
glomerulonephritis (Fig. 7.19).

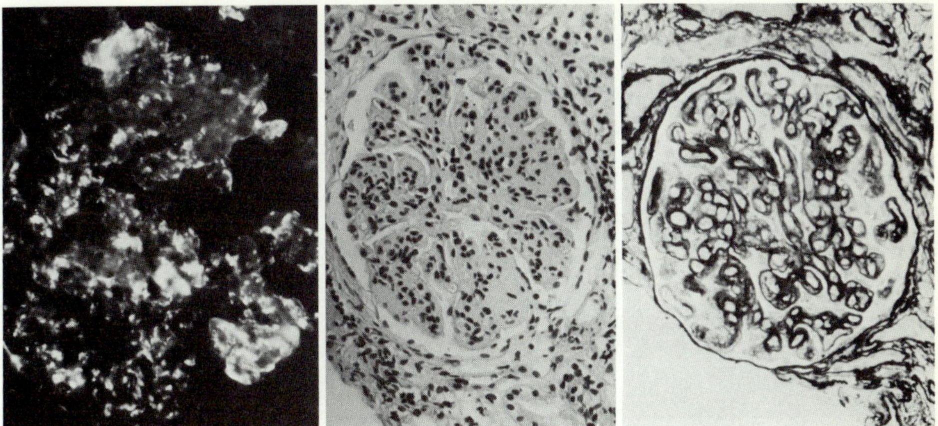

Figure 7.15. Glomerulus shows scattered deposits of C3. Larger aggregates at the glomerulus periphery. Mesangiocapillary glomerulonephritis.
Figure 7.16. Glomerulus lobulated with areas of hypercellularity and sclerosis in some lobules. Mesangiocapillary glomerulonephritis. H & E.
Figure 7.17. Glomerulus shows reduplication of basement membrane in a number of capillary loops. Mesangiocapillary glomerulonephritis. Methenamine silver.

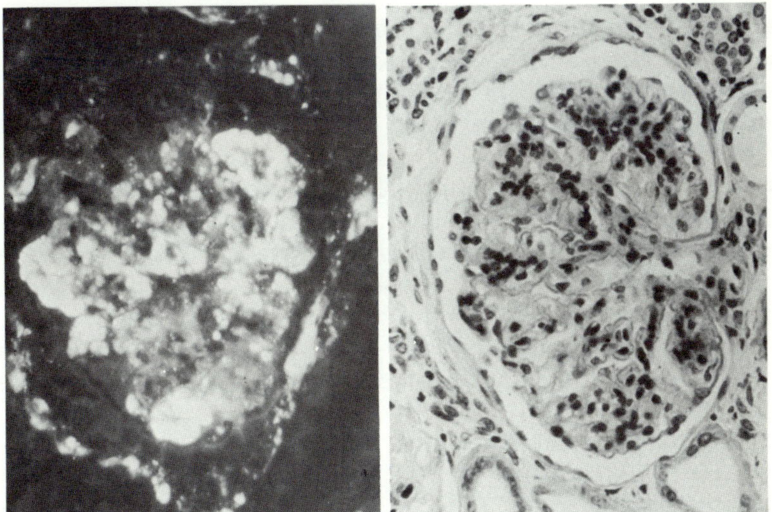

Figure 7.18. Glomerulus shows prominent lobulated aggregates of C3. Bowman's capsule also involved. Dense deposit disease.
Figure 7.19. Glomerulus shows lobulation with focal hypercellularity. Basement membrane of some capillary loops rather prominent. Dense deposit disease. PAS.

It is characterized on electron microscopy by segments of thickened darkly staining ribbon-like basement membranes.

C3NeF may be present in the serum and there is usually persisting hypocomplementaemia. Clinical presentation may be with nephritic or nephrotic syndromes.

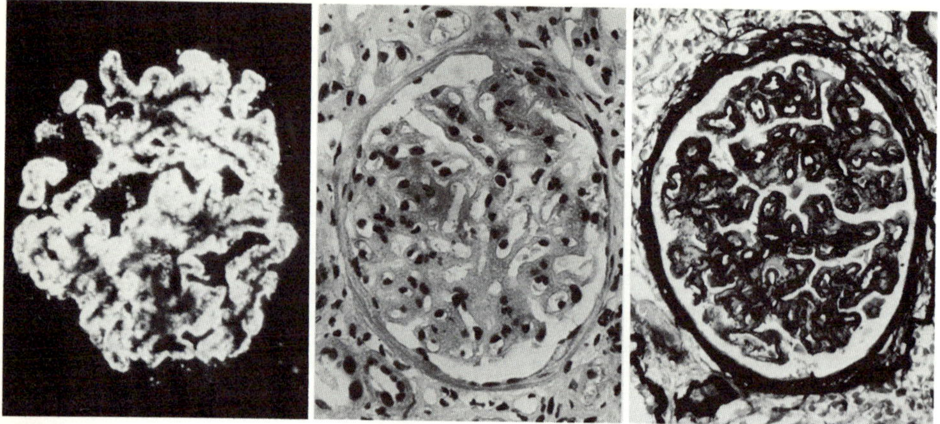

Figure 7.20. Glomerulus shows numerous speckled deposits of IgG in capillary loops. Membranous glomerulonephritis.
Figure 7.21. Glomerulus shows diffuse thickening of capillary loops. Membranous glomerulonephritis. H & E.
Figure 7.22. Glomerular basement membrane shows saw tooth appearance from projections of basement membrane between deposits. Membranous glomerulonephritis. Methenamine silver.

Idiopathic membranous glomerulonephritis

Glomeruli show granular deposits in loops (Fig. 7.20). IgG and C3 are usually conspicuous while IgA, IgM, C1q and C4 are present in varying degrees. The appearance may persist for many years with C1q diminishing. This condition has the characteristic fluorescence pattern of an immune-complex disease but the nature of the responsible antigens has not been identified.

On light microscopy, loops may show some thickening of the basement membrane (Fig. 7.21) and silver stains may reveal spikes of basement membrane material projecting between deposits (Fig. 7.22) particularly where the deposits are on the external aspect of the basement membrane.

Electron microscopy shows electron-dense deposits in the basement membrane (Fig. 7.23) and mesangium, corresponding to the staining seen with immunofluorescence.

Focal glomerulosclerosis

Large or small aggregates of IgM (Fig. 7.24) associated with C3 (Fig. 7.25) may be found in sclerotic segments. Glomeruli near the corticomedullary junction tend to be affected first. This may represent an immune complex process but the aetiology is obscure.

Histologically, segmental areas of sclerosis (Fig. 7.26) are usually seen when the disease presents and are commonly progressive, with steroid resistant proteinuria.

Goodpasture's syndrome (antiglomerular basement membrane disease)

Linear staining of glomerular basement membrane for IgG is characteristic

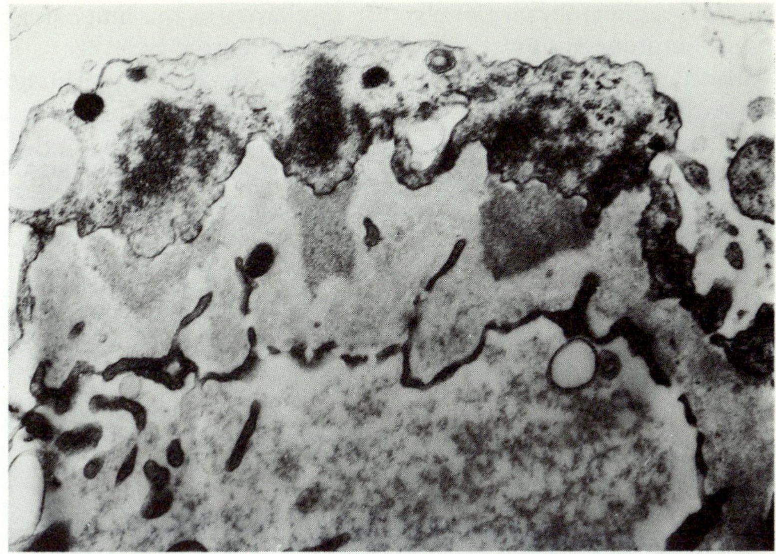

Figure 7.23. Electron micrograph shows deposits of electron-dense material within basement membrane of capillary loops. Membranous glomerulonephritis.

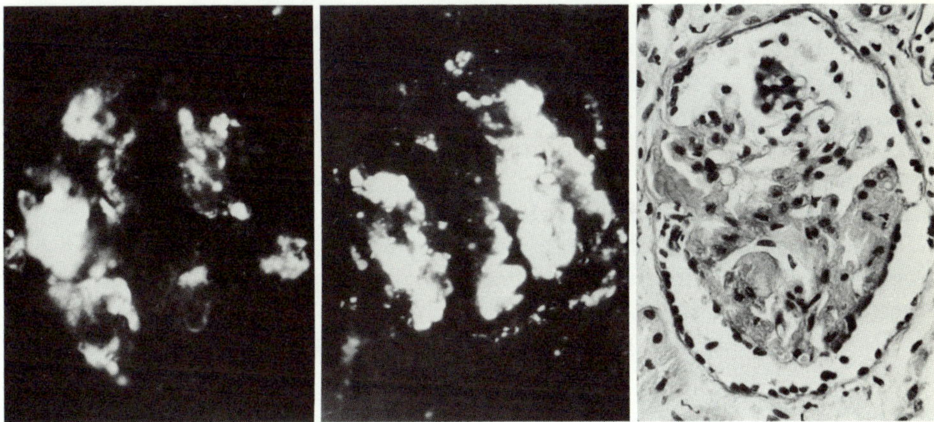

Figure 7.24. Glomerulus shows aggregates of IgM in sclerotic foci. Focal glomerulosclerosis.
Figure 7.25. Glomerulus shows prominent aggregates of C3 and smaller deposits in Bowman's capsule. Focal glomerulosclerosis.
Figure 7.26. Glomerulus shows prominent areas of sclerosis in several lobules. Focal glomerulosclerosis. H & E.

(Fig. 7.27). C3 does not usually parallel IgG staining and more commonly shows a segmental or granular pattern (Fig. 7.28).

Histologically the glomeruli may show crescent formation associated with fibrin deposition and glomerular destruction (Fig. 7.29).

Electron microscopy does not usually show clear evidence of antibody deposition.

The circulating antiglomerular basement membrane antibody cross-reacts with the basement membranes of alveolar capillaries in the lung, and plasma-pheresis and immune suppression help to reduce antibody levels.

Renal manifestations are frequently preceded by evidence of respiratory tract infections and it seems likely that this triggers off the formation of antibodies

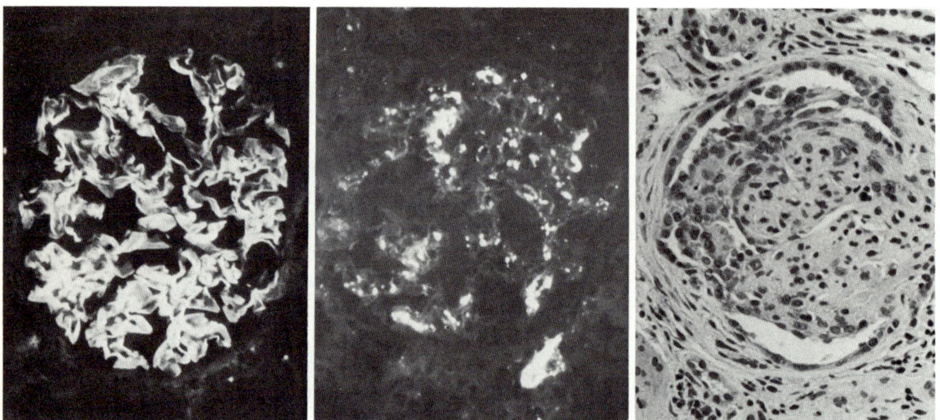

Figure 7.27. Glomerulus shows linear deposition of IgG in capillary loops. Goodpasture's syndrome.
Figure 7.28. Glomerulus shows specks of C3 and does not parallel IgG staining in Fig. 7.27. Goodpasture's syndrome.
Figure 7.29. Glomerulus shows marked damage with crescent formation. Cells lining Bowman's capsule are prominent. Goodpasture's syndrome. H & E.

cross-reacting with lung and kidney basement membranes. Antigens released from damaged tissues may reinforce the initial antigenic stimulus.

Rapidly progressive glomerulonephritis

When not associated with Goodpasture's syndrome, this condition may show granular deposits of immunoglobulins and complement. This appears to be an immune complex process, not necessarily poststreptococcal.

Histologically there is prominent crescent formation and fibrin deposition.

IgA nephropathy

The demonstration of IgA in the mesangium (Fig. 7.30) together with C3 and often some IgG points towards this diagnosis. Secretory IgA is not present in the glomerular lesions.

This appears to be a mesangiopathic process in which medium-sized immune complexes have been deposited in the mesangium. The prominence of IgA suggests a possible origin of immune complexes from mucosal areas in the alimentary or respiratory tracts.

Histologically there is usually mesangial proliferation with some expansion of mesangial matrix (Fig. 7.31).

Electron microscopy shows electron-dense deposits in the mesangium (Fig. 7.32).

Patients often present with haematuria sometimes following an upper respiratory infection.

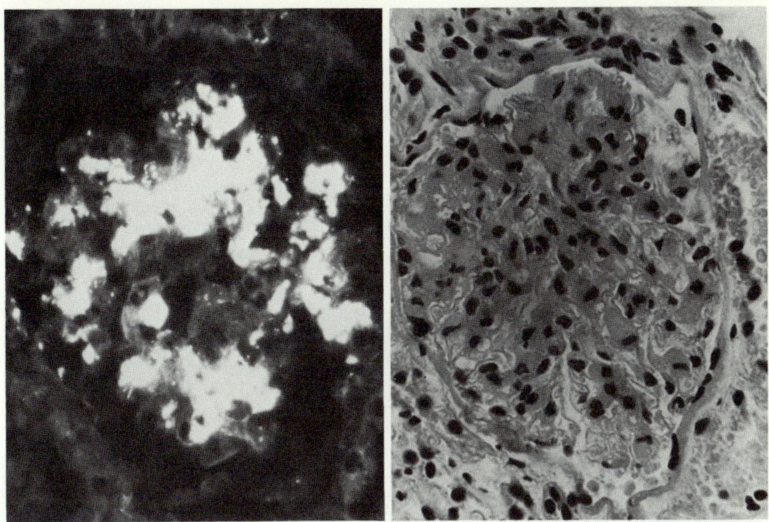

Figure 7.30. Glomerulus shows prominent mesangial aggregates of IgA. IgA nephropathy.
Figure 7.31. Glomerulus shows marked expansion of mesangial matrix by PAS-positive material. IgA nephropathy. PAS.

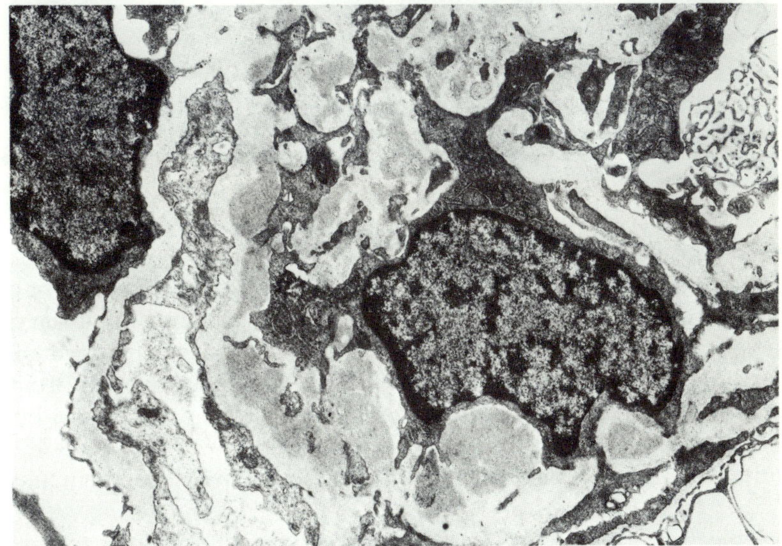

Figure 7.32. Electron micrograph shows prominent mesangial electron-dense deposits. IgA nephropathy.

Henoch Schönlein syndrome

IgA is often a significant component in the glomerular lesions and immunofluorescence appearances resemble those of IgA nephropathy. Fibrin may be present (Fig. 7.33).

Histologically the kidney usually shows a mesangioproliferative pattern (Fig. 7.34) but focal sclerosis and crescent formation can occur.

Although immunopathological appearances may be similar to IgA nephropathy the clinical symptoms are usually quite distinct. Patients are mostly children and have a skin rash and abdominal symptoms, sometimes associated with musculo-skeletal symptoms. Cryoglobulins have been found in about 60% of patients.

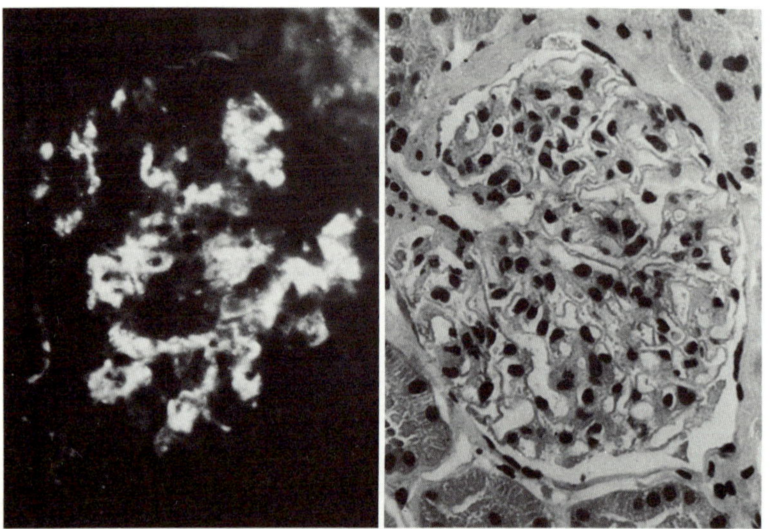

Figure 7.33. Glomerulus shows scattered mesangial aggregates of fibrin. Henoch-Schönlein syndrome.
Figure 7.34. Glomerulus shows some expansion of mesangial matrix. Henoch-Schönlein syndrome. H & E.

Systemic lupus erythematosus

Glomerular immunofluorescence appearances may vary from a diffuse granular pattern to a more irregular pattern with widespread deposits of varying size in mesangium and loops. In some glomeruli a mesangial pattern may predominate (Fig. 7.4). Although IgG and C3 predominate there is often a wide range of immunoglobulin and complement components present, and IgM, IgA, C1q, C4, fibrin and properdin may be identified.

Tubules may show granular deposits related to their basement membrane (Fig. 7.7).

Histologically, glomerular changes range from minimal to mesangioproliferative, diffuse proliferative and membranous. The diffuse proliferative pattern is particularly associated with subendothelial immune deposits and appears to be a more aggressive process than the other forms.

Electron microscopy reveals deposits in the mesangium and glomerular basement membrane as well as in relation to peritubular capillaries and tubular basement membrane.

Glomeruli may show widespread granular deposits on immunofluorescence (Fig. 7.35) in the presence of focal changes on light microscopy (Fig. 7.36). Electron microscopy confirms electron-dense deposits in the capillary basement membrane (Fig. 7.37) and mesangium.

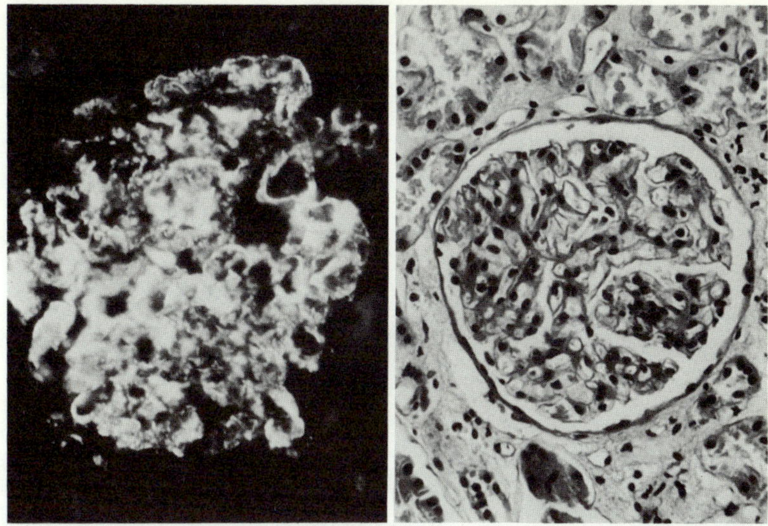

Figure 7.35. Glomerulus shows fine speckled deposits of IgG as well as larger aggregates within the mesangium. Systemic lupus erythematosus.

Figure 7.36. Glomerulus shows mesangial changes and some thick walled capillary loops. Systemic lupus erythematosus. H & E.

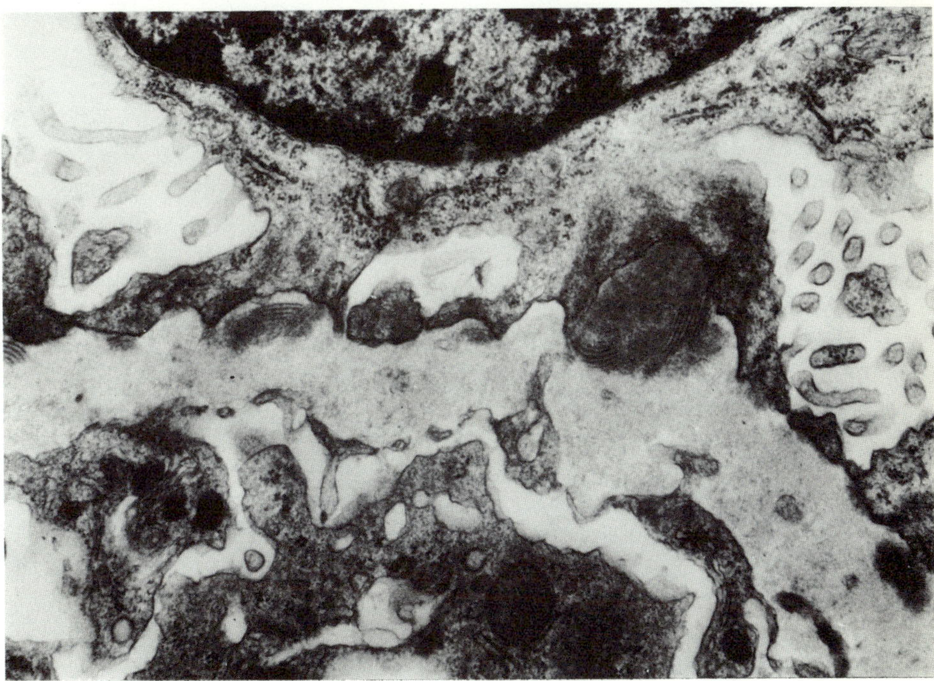

Figure 7.37. Electron micrograph shows subepithelial 'fingerprint' electron-dense deposits in basement membrane. Systemic lupus erythematosus.

Apparently confluent deposits can outline capillary loops on immuno-fluorescence (Fig. 7.38) and subendothelial deposits seen particularly in the diffuse proliferative form of lupus nephropathy (Fig. 7.39) can be demonstrated by electron microscopy (Fig. 7.40).

Circulating antinuclear antibodies against double-stranded DNA most closely parallel disease activity and the lodging of immune complexes containing anti-

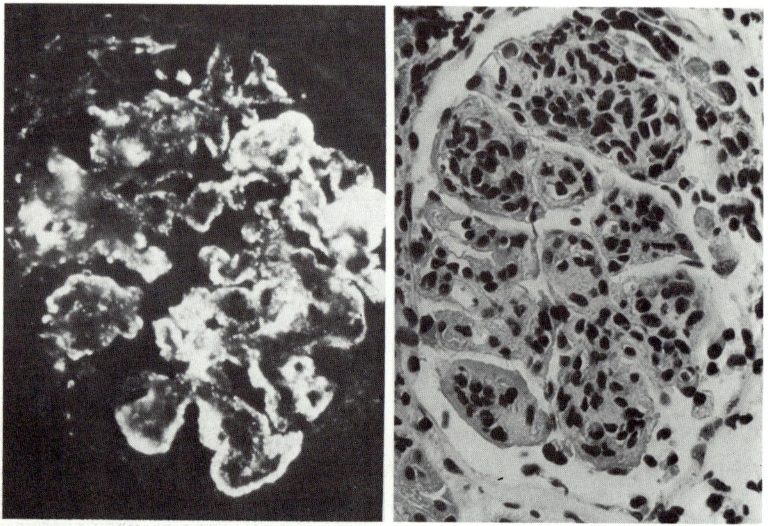

Figure 7.38. Capillary loops of glomerulus outlined by prominent C1q deposits. Systemic lupus erythematosus.
Figure 7.39. Glomerulus shows prominent lobulation and hypercellularity. Systemic lupus erythematosus. H & E.

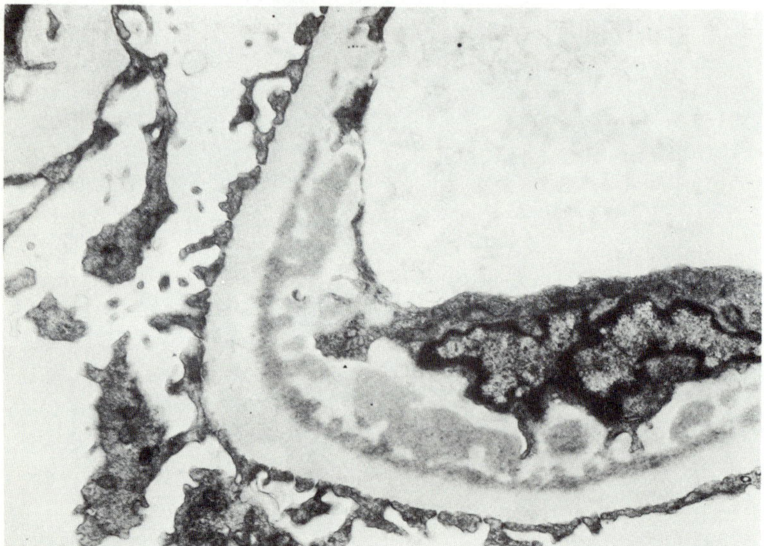

Figure 7.40. Electron micrograph showing subendothelial electron-dense deposits in capillary loop. Systemic lupus erythematosus.

bodies against nuclear antigens appears to be a significant pathogenic feature. Serum C3 and C4 are low and C3 may return to normal with treatment while a low C4 indicates persisting complement utilization.

Patients usually respond to immunosuppressive therapy. Plasmapheresis is sometimes used in a critical situation to reduce the level of circulating immune complexes.

Scleroderma

In many patients with scleroderma no plasma protein deposition is observed in the kidney. In other cases glomerular immunoglobulin and complement deposits may be seen, particularly in patients with antinuclear antibodies.

Histologically interlobular arteries show a distinctive subendothelial thickening by mucoid connective tissue. Areas of segmental necrosis and arteriolar fibrinoid change may be present in the terminal stage of the disease which is often associated with hypertension and renal failure.

Polyarteritis nodosa

Immune deposits are not usually present in glomeruli. Fibrin may be detected in glomerular lesions and affected vessels.

Histologically, in the microscopic form, interlobular arteries show a transmural inflammation, and afferent arterioles and segments of glomeruli may show fibrinoid necrosis.

Clinically this appears to be a multisystem disease associated with circulating immune complexes which lodge in medium-sized vessels rather than in capillaries. Hepatitis B antigen has a recognized association with this disease and may be a component of the immune complex.

Wegener's granulomatosis

The renal immunofluorescence findings are not specific. Glomeruli may show irregular aggregates of fibrin and variable immunoglobulin and complement deposition.

Histologically the kidneys show focal segmental proliferative and necrotizing lesions, often with the formation of crescents.

Diabetes mellitus

No specific immunofluorescence patterns occur. Sometimes irregular aggregates of immunoglobulins and complement may be found in glomerular lesions (Fig. 7.41). Glomeruli and tubules may show a linear pattern for IgG which appears to be due to non-immunological accumulation of protein in thickened basement membranes.

Histologically the glomeruli show a lobular pattern with central sclerotic areas surrounded by residual capillary loops as in the Kimmelstiel-Wilson lesion (Fig. 7.42), or a diffuse expansion of the mesangium and thickened capillary basement membrane as in diffuse glomerulosclerosis. Afferent and efferent arterioles show hyaline thickening. Interstitial nephritis and papillary necrosis may complicate the condition. The morphological appearances may sometimes resemble mesangiocapillary glomerulonephritis but can be

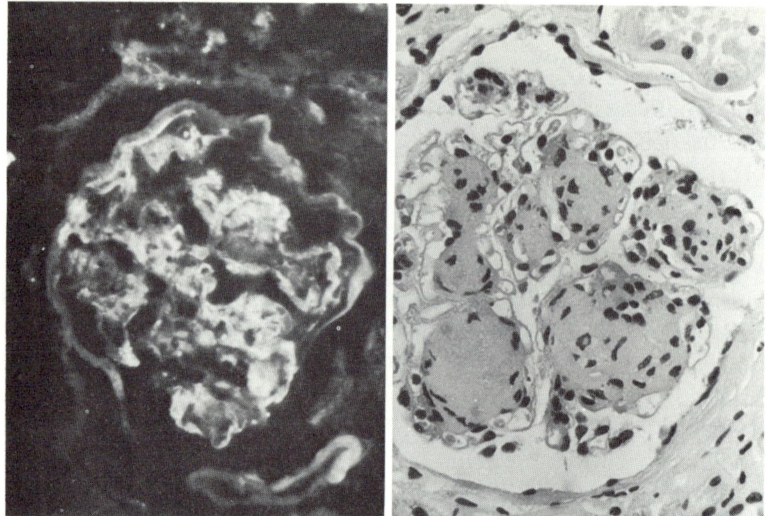

Figure 7.41. Glomerulus with Kimmelstiel-Wilson lesion shows patchy IgG deposition and some staining of Bowman's capsule. Diabetes mellitus.

Figure 7.42. Glomerulus shows marked lobulation with centrilobular sclerosis characteristic of Kimmelstiel-Wilson lesion. Diabetes mellitus. H & E.

distinguished by the metabolic features of diabetes and the absence of hypo-complementaemia and C3NeF.

Transplant kidney

Renal transplants may show a wide range of immunofluorescence appearances, some resulting from a recurrence of the original disease which led to the transplant while others may be a consequence of allograft rejection.

Recurrent glomerular lesions

These include dense deposit disease, mesangiocapillary glomerulonephritis, IgA nephropathy, Goodpasture's syndrome, focal sclerosing glomerulonephritis and to a lesser extent, membranous and lupus nephritis. Immunofluorescence findings in these conditions have been described earlier in this chapter.

Graft rejection

Immune complex deposition in glomeruli (Fig. 7.43) associated with a mesangial response (Fig. 7.44) may occur and staining of tubular basement membranes for immunoglobulins (Fig. 7.45) and complement is not unusual.

Histologically there are three patterns of graft rejection:

(*i*) The hyperacute form is associated with preformed antibodies against donor tissues and results in rapid thrombosis of major blood vessels and their branches.

(*ii*) The acute allograft rejection may occur a few days, weeks or months after the operation and recurrences can occur. The affected kidney shows interstitial oedema with mononuclear cell infiltration around tubules and peritubular

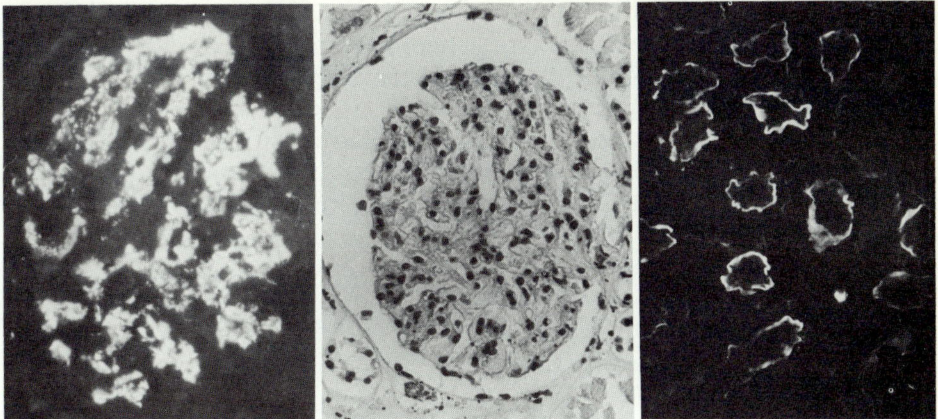

Figure 7.43. Transplanted kidney shows prominent mesangial deposits of IgM.
Figure 7.44. Glomerulus from same transplant kidney as Fig. 7.43 shows dilated congested capillary loops and mild mesangial response. H & E.
Figure 7.45. Basement membrane of tubules in transplant kidney stained with antiglobulin serum.

vessels (7.46). Antitubular basement membrane antibodies may be associated with this reaction, which is attributed mainly to host T lymphocytes reacting with the graft.

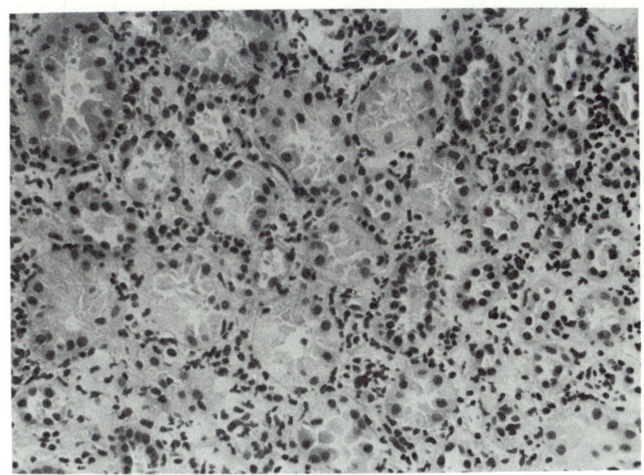

Figure 7.46. Tubules in same transplant kidney as Fig. 7.45 show degenerative changes with prominent interstitial mononuclear inflammatory cell infiltration. H & E.

(*iii*) In chronic graft rejection some months after the transplant occurred, arteries show prominent subendothelial thickening from intimal proliferation. Infarction can follow the occlusion of these vessels.

Interstitial nephritis
Tubular basement membranes may stain for immunoglobulins and complement. Interstitial nephritis is seen in a variety of conditions. It is now

recognized as an important consequence of allergic reactions to certain drugs. Methicillin is associated with interstitial nephritis and tubular basement membrane antibody production. Other penicillins, sulphonamides, phenindione, colistin, rifampicin and diphenylhydantoin may also cause an interstitial inflammatory reaction in the kidney. Interstitial nephritis is also associated with urinary tract infection and vesico-ureteric reflux.

Histologically there is interstitial infiltration of the kidney by inflammatory cells mainly mononuclear with varying degrees of tubular damage. In chronic pyelonephritis the process is patchy and leads to glomerular sclerosis and hypertensive changes in vessels.

No specific immunofluorescence findings are seen in chronic pyelonephritis. In chronic disease numerous tubular casts containing a variety of plasma proteins are present.

Multiple myeloma

Glomeruli do not usually show protein deposits. Tubules contain prominent casts. Although the myeloma protein may be monoclonal, the presence of a variety of immunoglobulins in the urine may result in casts staining with both anti-kappa and anti-lambda sera.

Amyloidosis

Usually glomeruli show no specific accumulation of plasma proteins. In some patients amyloid deposits may stain for monoclonal light chains.

Histologically there is a progressive deposition of amyloid in the mesangium and capillary loops in addition to variable deposits in interstitial tissues and blood vessels. The amyloid nature of the deposit is confirmed by special stains such as Congo Red and Thioflavine T.

Electron microscopy confirms the presence of amyloid fibrils with a diameter of approximately 800 nm and a periodicity of 500 nm.

Patients generally develop the nephrotic syndrome and claims to reverse the deposition of amyloid have not been sustained.

Haemolytic uraemic syndrome

Glomeruli show fibrin in capillary loops (Fig. 7.47) and in the lumen and walls of interstitial vessels.

Histologically, glomeruli may show areas of segmental necrosis and thrombi are conspicuous in glomeruli (Fig. 7.48), afferent arterioles and interlobular arteries.

This disease is mostly seen in infants and young children and is usually preceded by gastroenteritis or a respiratory tract infection which has precipitated intravascular coagulation.

IMMUNOPEROXIDASE METHOD

Immunoenzyme methods may be used as an alternative to immunofluorescence procedures to examine renal biopsy tissue. Horseradish peroxidase is substituted for the fluorescent label on the globulin fraction of antisera used for direct or

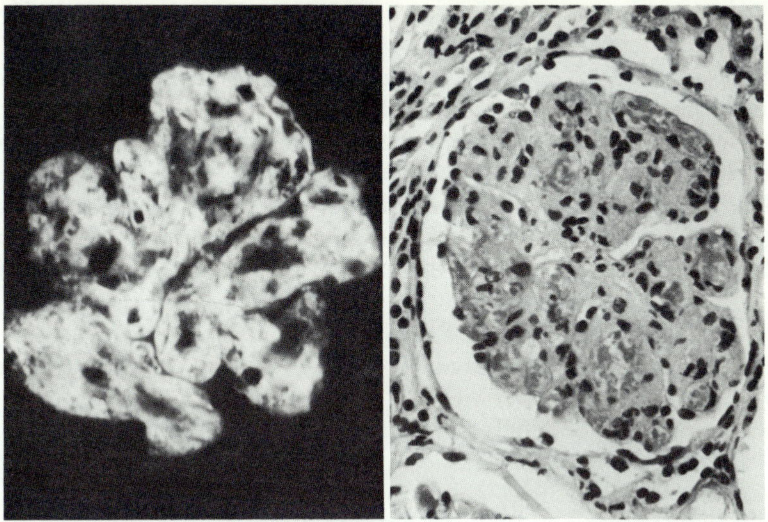

Figure 7.47. Glomerulus shows widespread deposition of fibrin. Haemolytic uraemic syndrome.
Figure 7.48. Glomerulus from same kidney as Fig. 7.47 showing patchy necrosis with neutrophil infiltration and some thrombi. H & E.

indirect staining and bridge techniques such as peroxidase bound by anti-peroxidase sera have been developed (Johnson et al, 1978).

The site of localization is demonstrated by treatment with 3,3′ diamino-benzidine tetrahydrochloride which, in the presence of hydrogen peroxide, is converted by peroxidase to a brown reaction product. This substance is un-affected by histological fixatives and processing, and is visible by light and electron microscopy; osmium postfixation further enhances ultrastructural identification.

Light microscopy

Direct staining techniques are frequently complicated by non-specific staining which appears to be less in the indirect and bridge methods. The reader con-templating the use of peroxidase for light microscopy is advised to consider the unlabelled antibody immunoperoxidase technique (Elias & Miller, 1975) which has been successfully applied to the study of renal biopsies and permits the use of a variety of counterstains.

Electron microscopy

Immunoperoxidase methods have been used extensively for ultrastructural studies concerned with determining the nature of immune deposits.

Reagents

(*i*) *1% (w/v) formaldehyde.* Prepare a fresh 2% solution by stirring 2 g paraformaldehyde in distilled water at 80°C and make up to 100 ml. For use, dilute in an equal volume of double strength cacodylate buffer.

(*ii*) *Cacodylate buffer.* 0.1M sodium cacodylate, 0.14M sucrose, 4 mM Ca^{++}, pH 7.3.

(*iii*) *30% (w/v) sucrose solution.* 30 g sucrose in 70 ml distilled water made up to 100 ml.

(*iv*) *Saturated sucrose solution.* Stir sucrose in warm distilled water until no further sucrose dissolves, and cool to 4°C.

(*v*) *Peroxidase-labelled antisera.* These are available commercially or the globulin fraction of the required antiserum may be labelled with horseradish peroxidase (Sigma type 4) by the method of Nakane & Kawaoi (1974).

(*vi*) *1% (v/v) hydrogen peroxide.* Stock solution comprises 100 vol hydrogen peroxide, 30% w/v. Add 1 vol stock solution to 29 vol cacodylate buffer immediately before use.

(*vii*) *Diaminobenzidine reagent.* Prepare a fresh solution by dissolving 25 mg 3,3′ diaminobenzidine tetrahydrochloride (*N.B.* this is a potent carcinogen) in 25 ml 0.1 M cacodylate buffer pH 7.3. Filter through Whatman No 1 paper and place in dark. Immediately before use add 1 ml 1% hydrogen peroxide to 24 ml staining reagent and mix.

(*viii*) *Toluidine blue.* Stock solution comprises 1% toluidine blue in 1% aqueous borax. Dilute 1 in 20 with distilled water for use.

(*ix*) *2.5% (v/v) glutaraldehyde.* 10 ml 25% aqueous ultrastructural grade glutaraldehyde in 40 ml double strength cacodylate buffer and 50 ml distilled water.

(*x*) *1% (v/v) buffered osmium tetroxide.* Stock solution comprises 2% osmium in distilled water. Add equal vol double strength cacodylate buffer.

Method

Tissue preparation. Prefix a 1 mm cube of fresh tissue in 1% formaldehyde for 1 h. Wash twice in cacodylate buffer and once in 30% sucrose. Soak tissue in 30% sucrose for 30 min at 4°C. Snap-freeze tissue block in liquid nitrogen and place on chuck in cryokit at −60°C. Cut sections with a hand held razor blade and collect on a drop of saturated sucrose. Stain an early section with toluidine blue to determine position of glomeruli and trim block accordingly. Cut further sections and transfer to drops of cacodylate buffer in separate wells of flat bottomed microculture plates (Cook M29AR).

Staining (direct). Add 25 μl of appropriate peroxidase-labelled antiserum to each well, cover plate and leave for 30 min at room temperature. Carefully aspirate antiserum and wash tissue × 3 by flooding wells with cacodylate buffer and aspirating. Postfix tissue for 30 min in 2.5% glutaraldehyde. Aspirate glutaraldehyde and wash × 3 with cacodylate buffer. Add diaminobenzidine reagent and incubate in the dark for 30 min. Aspirate reagent from well and wash × 3 with cacodylate buffer.

Processing for electron microscopy. Postfix with 1% buffered osmium tetroxide for 30 min, wash in cacodylate buffer for 30 min and dehydrate through acetone series—25%, 75% and 95% each for 5 min and 100% twice for 5 min. Infiltrate tissue with 50% Spurr's resin in acetone for 30 min followed by 100% Spurr's resin. Embed flat in Balzer's moulds in fresh Spurr's resin polymerized overnight at 60°C. For section cutting on the ultramicrotome the resin block is orientated so that the tissue is on edge and sections present two external faces which have been exposed to the reagents and a central core which has not been penetrated and remains unstained.

Controls include tissue treated with peroxidase-labelled normal serum and tissues which have not been exposed to labelled serum.

Comments

Immunoperoxidase methods for light microscopy permit the use of counter-stains, do not require a fluorescence microscope and sections may be stored as a permanent record for future reference.

Disadvantages of immunoperoxidase staining are that what is essentially a one stage immunofluorescence method is replaced by a longer multistage procedure which in general is less well standardized and uses more expensive reagents.

I have personally never found that the various shades of brown obtained with peroxidase match the clarity of the brilliant fluorescence obtained with the standard FITC-labelled antisera. Provided the observer is motivated to record significant results on film the absence of a permanent preparation is not a particular disadvantage. Storage of the original block when adequate tissue remains permits further examination of the tissue.

The undisputed advantage of immunoperoxidase staining is for ultra-structural studies of immune deposits. Problems include the requirement to maintain antigenicity and yet preserve ultrastructural architecture which is easily distorted when tissues have been frozen and exposed to antisera and other reagents. A particular problem is the limited degree of penetration obtained with the proxidase labelled antiserum when attempting to identify antigens within tissues, in contrast to antigens which are readily accessible on the surfaces of cells or membranes. Our method using the microtitre plate conserves reagents and permits both faces of the tissue section to be stained as well as making embedding and sectioning easier than in most other methods.

While some may advocate the use of immunoperoxidase staining as a substitute for immunofluorescence, in practice immunofluorescence has been proved to be a well standardized procedure accepted widely in routine laboratories. Immunoperoxidase studies in our laboratory are largely reserved for research investigations at the ultrastructural level.

EXTRA-RENAL INVESTIGATIONS

Skin biopsy

Immunofluorescence examination of the skin may facilitate diagnosis of renal disease. If skin lesions are present it is best to take a biopsy of affected and unaffected areas. Each sample is bisected, one portion being placed in normal saline for immunofluorescence, the other in formalin for histopathological examination. The immunofluorescence biopsy is snap-frozen and embedded in the same way as a renal biopsy and about 15 sections are cut. Paragon-stained sections at the beginning and end of the series are examined to ensure the presence of epidermis and dermis. Sections are stained with FITC antisera directed against IgG, IgA, IgM, IgE, C3, Clq, C4, albumin, fibrin, and properdin. Sections are washed twice and mounted as for renal biopsies.

Staining of the dermal-epidermal junction
Skin from patients with systemic lupus erythematosus may show dermal-epidermal staining for IgG, IgM, IgA and C3. This is usually granular (Fig. 7.49) but sometimes appears linear. Staining is frequently found in clinically

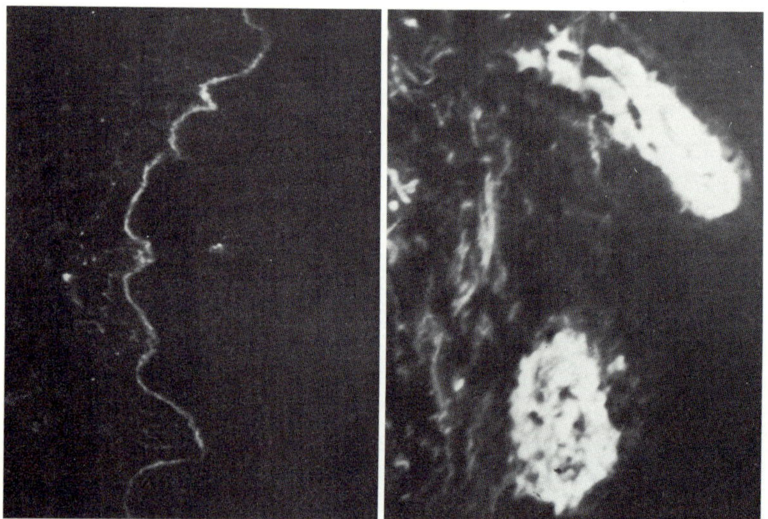

Figure 7.49. Skin biopsy shows deposition of IgM at dermal-epidermal junction. Systemic lupus erythematosus.
Figure 7.50. Skin biopsy shows fibrin deposition in walls and lumen of dermal vessels. Polyarteritis nodosa.

unaffected as well as in affected areas of skin. In discoid lupus, which is not usually associated with renal disease, staining is restricted to the area of the skin lesion. It has been suggested that in some patients the discoid form may progress to the systemic form.

Wertheimer & Barland (1976) evaluated the significance of the lupus band test in 53 patients. The test was positive on normal skin in 45%, of whom half had active renal disease.

Vascular staining
IgA is seen in the walls of dermal vessels of some patients with IgA nephropathy. This should not be confused with the granular IgA dermal-epidermal staining of the papillary dermis in patients with dermatitis herpetiformis.

In polyarteritis nodosa, dermal vessel walls and immediate surroundings show conspicuous fibrin (Fig. 7.50) and other plasma proteins.

Lung biopsy
Lung tissue is of particular interest when a patient is suspected of having antiglomerular basement membrane disease and a diagnosis of Goodpasture's

syndrome is being considered. Lung tissue is embedded in OCT as for kidney, and frozen sections are treated with antisera in the same manner. Patients with Goodpasture's syndrome show linear staining of the alveolar capillary walls for immunoglobulin, usually IgG and complement, particularly C3. This test may help to distinguish Goodpasture's syndrome from other conditions where glomerulonephritis may be associated with lung haemorrhage.

ELUTION STUDIES

From time to time a laboratory may have access to a kidney specimen from a case of immune-complex disease of uncertain aetiology in which associated features suggest a possible antigen source and the laboratory is invited to make further investigations. Acid citrate buffer pH 3.4 (15 ml 0.1M citric acid, 5 ml 0.1M sodium citrate and 0.85 g sodium chloride made up to 100 ml with distilled water) dissociates immune complexes so that antibody may be released and antigen in the kidney made accessible to detection by specific antisera. The eluted antibody may be concentrated and its specific activity determined by immunofluorescence on appropriate antigen preparations. Elution techniques can be applied to frozen sections but clearly a greater yield of antibody will be eluted if a larger sample of kidney is available. Glomeruli can be isolated from kidney cortex and such preparations avoid the criticism that any antibody detected in the eluate has come from a non-glomerular site. Control preparations are treated with phosphate-buffered saline, pH 7.1.

Such studies should be considered when the patient has a recognized auto-immune disease. The appropriate autoantibody can be tested against biopsy material as an antigen detector. Alternatively specific antibody can be obtained from resected material isolated from the patient. It is important to appreciate that the antigen in the glomerular lesion is usually well masked by antibody and partial elution of antibody is often required to enable detection of the antigen.

REFERENCES

Elias J M, Miller F 1975 A comparison of the unlabelled enzyme method with immunofluorescence for the evaluation of human immunologic renal disease. American Journal of Clinical Pathology 64: 464–471
Johnson G D, Holborow E J, Dorling J 1978 Immunofluorescence and immunoenzyme techniques. In: Handbook of Experimental Immunology ed Weir D M 3rd edn. vol 1: ch 15, p 15.22–15.28 Blackwell, Oxford
Lachmann P J, Hobart M J 1978 Complement technology. In: Handbook of Experimental Immunology ed Weir D M 3rd edn. vol 1: ch 5A Blackwell, Oxford
McGiven A R, Hunt J S, Day W A, Bailey R R 1978 Tamm-Horsfall protein in the glomerular capsular space. Journal of Clinical Pathology 31: 620–625
Nairn R C 1976. Fluorescent Protein Tracing. 4th edn. Churchill Livingstone, Edinburgh
Nakane P K, Kawaoi A 1974 Peroxidase-labelled antibody. A new method of conjugation. The Journal of Histochemistry and Cytochemistry 22: 1084–1091
Wertheimer D, Barland P 1976 Clinical significance of immune deposits in the skin in SLE. Arthritis and Rheumatism 19: 1249–1255

UNCITED BIBLIOGRAPHY

Cameron J S, Glasgow E F, Ogg C S, White R H R 1970 Membranoproliferative glomerulonephritis and persistent hypocomplementaemia. British Medical Journal 4: 7–14

Churg J, Grishman E 1975 Ultrastructure of glomerular disease: A review. Kidney International 7: 254–270

Germuth F G, Rodriguez E 1975 Focal mesangiopathic glomerulonephritis: Prevalence and pathogenesis. Kidney International 7: 216–223

Heptinstall R H 1974 Pathology of the Kidney. 2nd edn. Little Brown, Boston

Heptinstall R H 1976 Interstitial nephritis. A brief review. American Journal of Pathology 83: 214–236

Jenis E H, Lowenthal D T 1977 Kidney Biopsy Interpretation. Davis, Philadelphia

Meadows R 1978 Renal Histopathology: A Light, Electron and Immunofluorescent Microscopy Study of Renal Disease. 2nd edn Oxford University Press, Oxford

Turner D R, Wilson D M, Lake A, Heaton J M, Leibowitz S, Cameron J S 1979 An evaluation of the immunoperoxidase technique in renal biopsy diagnosis. Clinical Nephrology 11: 13–17

West C D 1976 Pathogenesis and approaches to therapy of membranoproliferative glomerulonephritis. Kidney International 9: 1–7

Wilson C B 1977 Recent advances in the immunological aspects of renal disease. Federation Proceedings 36: 2171–2175

Wilson C B, Dixon F J 1974 Diagnosis of immunopathologic renal disease. Kidney International 5: 389–401

8
Transplantation
A. R. McGiven

Renal transplantation is acceptable treatment for many patients with chronic renal failure, particularly those in younger age groups. The renal failure may be due to a congenital disorder like polycystic disease or acquired conditions such as glomerulonephritis, pyelonephritis or analgesic nephropathy. The nature of the disease is important because some disorders such as glomerulonephritis may recur in the transplanted organ. In addition the transplanted kidney may be affected by allograft rejection unless it has been donated by an identical twin.

Before transplantation, immunological techniques are employed to determine the blood group and tissue type of the donor and recipient and also to study the compatibility between the donor's lymphocytes and the recipient's serum.

After transplantation the immunological status of the recipient of the graft is studied with a view to predicting and monitoring allograft rejection episodes and their control by immunosuppressive agents.

HLA ANTIGENS

It is believed that, at least in part, the rejection of an organ graft results from stimulation of the immunological system of the host by antigens present in the donor tissue which the host does not possess. In man, the major histocompatibility complex which controls the presence or absence of transplantation antigens is called the HLA region and is located on chromosome 6. Four genetic loci have so far been identified, called HLA-A, HLA-B, HLA-C and HLA-D. Most work has been carried out on the identification of HLA-A and HLA-B antigens and it has been observed that accelerated rejection of a graft occurs in the presence of antibodies in the donor against these specific antigens. B lymphocytes have a series of antigens apparently determined by the HLA-D locus. Mixed lymphocyte culture distinguishes these antigens and B lymphocyte typing by conventional microcytotoxicity is now being used in some laboratories.

HLA antigens are glycoproteins on the surface membrane of most nucleated cells and the lymphocyte is an accessible and suitable cell for histocompatibility typing.

Many antigens have been detected but in some instances cross-reactivity between certain antigens sometimes makes their discrimination difficult. Where a particular antigen is not yet well defined it is distinguished by prefix w before its numeral. Table 8.1 lists HLA antigens.

Table 8.1. HLA antigens

A locus	B locus	C locus	D locus
HLA-A1	HLA-B5	HLA-Cw1	HLA-Dw1
HLA-A2	HLA-B7	HLA-Cw2	HLA-Dw2
HLA-A3	HLA-B8	HLA-Cw3	HLA-Dw3
HLA-A9	HLA-B12	HLA-Cw4	HLA-Dw4
HLA-A10	HLA-B13	HLA-Cw5	HLA-Dw5
HLA-A11	HLA-B14	HLA-Cw6	HLA-Dw6
HLA-Aw23	HLA-B15		HLA-Dw7
HLA-Aw24	HLA-Bw16		
HLA-A25	HLA-B17		
HLA-A26	HLA-B18		
HLA-A28	HLA-Bw21		
HLA-A29	HLA-Bw22		
HLA-Aw30	HLA-B27		
HLA-Aw31	HLA-Bw35		
HLA-Aw32	HLA-B37		
HLA-Aw33	HLA-Bw38		
HLA-Aw34	HLA-Bw39		
HLA-Aw36	HLA-B40		
HLA-Aw43	HLA-Bw41		
	HLA-Bw42		

HISTOCOMPATIBILITY INVESTIGATION

TISSUE TYPING

Equipment

Terasaki 60 well tissue typing trays—Test tubes 12×75 mm—Multiple dispenser—Hamilton microsyringes: $50 \mu l$; $100 \mu l$; $250 \mu l$—Centrifuge—Inverted phase-contrast microscope.

Reagents

Tissue typing antisera—Mineral oil—Ficoll-Conray separating medium—0.9% saline—Veronal buffer pH 7.2 (Oxoid C.F. diluent)—5% eosin—Rabbit complement—20% neutral formalin.

Antisera with selective specificity against known HLA antigens are used in a complement-dependent microcytotoxicity assay to type lymphocytes from donor and recipient.

Sera for typing are acquired from a variety of sources including blood donors, particularly multiparous women. Such sera are screened against a panel of lymphocytes containing a variety of HLA types and highly reactive and specific sera are retained for the tissue typing panel. Sera may be collected and stored in aliquots at $-70°C$ or freeze-dried. In typing for renal transplants much attention has been paid to the HLA-A and HLA-B systems on preparations of whole lymphocytes, but it is likely that in future more attention will be given to B lymphocyte typing and the HLA-D system.

For use, strongly reactive sera may be diluted until they are still able to produce a 4+ reading. It is usual to use three sera when testing for a particular HLA antigen.

Method

Preparation of trays. 60 test tubes containing the typing antisera are set up in a carrier that holds six across, spaced at the same distance as the wells in the Terasaki trays. A batch of similar trays can be prepared using a multiple dispenser which is rinsed ten times between each row of six sera. A negative control of human AB serum and a positive control of antilymphocyte serum may be added to each tray. Add $1-2\,\mu l$ of mineral oil to each well in the Terasaki tray to prevent evaporation of serum, and then using the multiple dispenser add $1\,\mu l$ of each test serum to the wells in the trays. Trays may then be covered and stored frozen at $-30°C$ or below.

Collection of specimen. Collect 5 ml sterile clotted blood and an unclotted sample of 3 ml blood in a sterile tube containing 0.3 ml of 5% EDTA. Samples are stored at room temperature. The clotted sample is used for ABO and Rh grouping as well as hepatitis BsAg and any other serology.

Separation medium. A variety of media are available for the separation of lymphocytes by differential centrifugation. The method described here employs Ficoll-Conray which is prepared by dissolving 1 g Ficoll powder in 13.8 ml distilled water and mixing with 2.6 ml Conray 280 (May & Baker). The medium should be protected from the light once made up and can be used for a few days. Alternatively Ficoll-Hypaque may be used (*see* Mixed Lymphocyte Culture).

Preparation of lymphocyte suspension.

(*i*) To a 12×75 mm test tube, add 0.4 ml EDTA blood sample, 1.4 ml 0.9% saline, and 0.6 ml Ficoll-Conray separation medium carefully to bottom of tube to form a layer.

(*ii*) Centrifuge at $400\,g$ for 10 min and harvest lymphocytes from the Ficoll-saline interface.

(*iii*) Wash twice with veronal buffer (pH 7.2), centrifuging at $180\,g$ for 3 min on each occasion.

(*iv*) Decant the buffer after the last wash, and resuspend to 2000 cell/μl.

Tissue typing procedure.

(*i*) Add $1\,\mu l$ of the lymphocyte suspension to each well of the 60 well Terasaki tissue typing tray which has been preprimed with antisera.

(*ii*) Incubate at room temperature for 30 min.

(*iii*) Add $5\,\mu l$ rabbit complement to each well.

(*iv*) Incubate at room temperature for 60 min.

(*v*) Add $2\,\mu l$ 5% eosin to each well.

(*vi*) Incubate at room temperature for 2 min.

(*vii*) Add $1\,\mu l$ 20% neutral formalin.

(*viii*) Leave to settle for 20 min.

(*ix*) Read.

Direct WBC crossmatch

This test is used to determine the compatibility of the donor's lymphocytes and the recipient's serum and can be used either to find the most favourable donor for a given patient or to find the most suitable recipient to receive a transplant from a specific donor. A direct match tray is prepared in which sera from prospective recipients have been added and arranged according to ABO blood group. The donor's lymphocytes prepared as above are added to each well and the same procedures as for tissue typing are carried out.

Reading

Tissue type and direct match trays are read on an inverted phase-contrast microscope and results are scored according to the percentage kill of lymphocytes. Live cells appear as bright well-defined refractile bodies. Dead cells absorb the eosin and stain darkly. Flooding the wells with buffer may improve the clarity of the cells for reading the microcytotoxicity test:

Score	0	1	2	3	4	5
% kill	0–10	11–30	31–50	51–70	71–100	unreadable

A significant level of cytotoxicity must be assessed against the background given by a variety of sera, and readings of 1 and 2 are usually not significant. Select the pair of alleles which give the strongest reaction in each HLA group tested. Sometimes it is only possible to detect one allele by this test. This may indicate a homozygous state, absence of appropriate antisera or cross-reactive antigens.

Selection of suitable recipient or donor

(*i*) ABO blood group compatibility.

(*ii*) Direct match compatibility.

(*iii*) Closeness of tissue type. In this regard the B locus appears to be more important. It is better to have 2 HLA-A mismatches than 1 HLA-B locus mismatch.

(*iv*) Presence of antibodies in the recipient providing direct match is compatible.

At first sight it seems strange that the presence of HLA antibodies in the recipient could be a positive factor in the selection for a transplant. Such patients have usually received blood transfusions (or dialysis). It is possible that the antibodies exert a protective blocking effect but the mechanism responsible for beneficial effects of transfusion is unknown (van Rood et al 1978).

B lymphocyte typing

Typing of B lymphocytes is not yet a routine procedure but is likely to become so. It is carried out on B cell enriched preparations where T cells have been removed by the sedimentation of rosettes formed by T cells with neuraminadase-treated sheep erythrocytes.

The microcytotoxicity test is conducted as for HLA-A and HLA-B typing except that cells are incubated with antisera at 37°C to avoid confusion with cold reacting autoantibodies. As B cells appear to be more resistant to cytolysis than T cells, B cells are incubated with antibody for 1 h and then with complement for 2 h. *See* Terasaki et al (1978) for detailed methods.

Significance of B lymphocyte antibodies

Although transplant recipients with cytotoxic antibodies against donor lymphocytes risk developing hyperacute rejection, some patients with antibodies against B cells have not experienced such episodes (Lobo et al, 1977). It has been suggested that the presence of cold reacting autoantibodies against B cells may even have an enhancing effect on the transplant while warm reacting allo-antibodies may be associated with accelerated rejection (Terasaki et al, 1978). Clearly tissue typing laboratories will be paying closer attention to B cell anti-bodies in the future and cross-matching may be performed against B and T donor lymphocytes.

MIXED LYMPHOCYTE CULTURE

When lymphocytes from two individuals are cultured together some of the cells react by undergoing blast transformation. The degrees of proliferation may be measured by the incorporation of tritiated thymidine into the DNA of the dividing cells. For the one way reaction, DNA synthesis in one population is inhibited by treatment with mitomycin C, thus enabling the response of the other population to be measured.

This test may be used to assess the compatibility between potential donors and a recipient for a renal transplant. It is probably most useful when screening prospective donors from within the family of the recipient. As the test requires six days to perform it cannot be applied in a prospective manner to the selection of donors where cadaveric grafts are concerned. This may become possible with primed LD typing (Sheehy & Bach, 1976).

Equipment
All glassware and reagents must be sterile.

Universal containers 30 ml—Glass pipette 10 ml—Conical flask 100 ml—Pasteur pipettes—Centrifuge tubes, graduated 10 ml conical polypropylene—Neubauer counting chamber and Dahl pipette—Plastic microculture trays, 96 wells, round bottomed with lids—Centrifuge for $200g$ and $400g$ or $1250g$—Multiple cell harvester—Scintillation counter—Roto-torque rotator.

Reagents
Ethylenediaminetetraacetic acid (EDTA). Weigh 2.7 g EDTA—Dissolve in 100 ml distilled water to give 2.7% solution—Add 0.75 ml to universals and sterilize (for 15 ml blood)—Add 1.5 ml to universal containers and sterilize (for 30 ml blood).

Dulbecco's phosphate-buffered saline (pH 7.3, PBS). Assemble clean glass screw-topped bottles capable of holding 200 ml; avoid perished rubber lid liners—Measure 200 ml distilled water into each bottle—Add two Dulbecco A tablets to each bottle—Screw down lid loosely, cover lid with tinfoil and sterilize in autoclave on slow exhaust setting to prevent explosion—Allow bottles to cool, tighten lids, label with date and store at 4°C.

Ficoll-Hypaque density gradient (density 1.077 g/ml). Weigh out 18 g of Ficoll directly into 200 ml stoppered measuring cylinder—Add approximately 180 ml distilled water—Dissolve Ficoll by shaking for about 30 min—Make solution up to 200 ml when fully dissolved and remove 8 ml, leaving 182 ml of 9%

Ficoll—Pipette 54.5 ml 50% Hypaque into measuring cylinder and make up to 80 ml with distilled water, to make a 33.9% solution—Mix together 182 ml 9% Ficoll and 80 ml 33.9% Hypaque—Aliquot 8 ml quantities into plastic universals. Autoclave. Store frozen. Avoid exposure to light.

Ammonium chloride solution. Dissolve 0.829 g NH_4Cl and 0.1 g $NaHCO_3$ in 100 ml distilled water. Autoclave.

Acetic acid (2.5%) cell counting diluent. Add 625 μl of concentrated acetic acid to 25 ml distilled water and mix.

Mitomycin C. Prepare a solution containing 1 mg mytomycin C per ml PBS. Store in 1 ml aliquots at $-20°C$.

Hepes buffer. Weigh 23.831 g of Hepes powder in 100 ml beaker—Using funnel, transfer to 100 ml volumetric flask—Make up to 100 ml with sterile distilled water—Dissolve powder with stirring—Transfer to screw-topped bottle, label and autoclave.

Eagles minimum essential medium (EMEM) supplemented for MLC. 10 ml EMEM ($\times 10$ conc)—10 ml human AB serum heat-inactivated at 56°C for 30 min—2 ml sodium bicarbonate (CO_2 saturated) 4.4% containing phenol red indicator (Wellcome)—1.25 ml Hepes—1.0 ml L. glutamine—0.025 ml gentamycin (40 mg/ml)—0.5 ml penicillin (10 000 u/ml)—0.5 ml streptomycin (10 000 μg/ml—75 ml sterile deionized water—Make up to 100 ml in sterile containers and store at 4°C. (RPMI 1640 medium enhances thymidine counts but is more expensive.)

Scintillation counting fluid. 5.5 g, 2,5 diphenyloxazole—0.1 g 1,4-bis [2(4-methyl-5-phenyloxazolyl)] benzene in 1 litre of toluene.—Toluene may be re-methyl-5-phenyloxazolyl)] benzene in 1 litre toluene—Toluene may be re-distilled when background counts become too high—Fresh scintillants must be added after distillation.

6-³H thymidine 5Ci/mM (Amersham, TRA 61).

Method

Collection of specimen. The results of a recent total and differential white blood cell count should be available so that a sample of appropriate size is collected. For donors with a normal white blood count calculate a minimum yield at 1×10^6 lymphocytes per ml whole blood. Collect 15 ml blood from donors into EDTA in sterile containers (0.5 ml 2.7% EDTA/10 ml blood) and label each clearly; it is essential not to confuse related donors. At the same time a sample should be collected for total white cell count and differential.

Separation of lymphocytes. Using a bulb attached to a sterile glass pipette, transfer 10 ml of the anticoagulated blood into a sterile conical flask. Add 20 ml of Dulbecco's phosphate buffer (PBS), taking care to flame the neck of the bottle, cap and mix. Other volumes may be used but the ratio of 1 vol blood to 2 vol PBS should be maintained. Carefully layer the diluted blood onto 8 ml sterile Ficoll-Hypaque solution in a universal container held at 45° to prevent mixing. Centrifuge the universal at 400 g for 45 min or 1250 g for 20 min. Using a sterile pasteur pipette carefully remove the cloudy interface which contains lymphocytes, and add to a sterile universal containing 5 ml PBS at room temperature. Care should be taken not to aspirate cells from within the Ficoll-Hypaque gradient as this contains polymorphonuclear cells. Wash cells by centrifugation at 200 g for 10 min. Discard supernatant. Resuspend lymphocytes in 5 ml PBS and transfer to sterile plastic centrifuge tube. Centrifuge again at 200 g for 10 min and discard supernatant.

Mixed lymphocyte culture procedure. Treat cell pellet with 0.83% NH_4Cl solution, several times if necessary, to eliminate red cell contamination—Add 5 ml NH_4Cl and resuspend cells—Incubate in waterbath at 37°C for 5–10 min—Centrifuge at 200 g for 10 min and aspirate NH_4Cl—Wash cells with PBS; three PBS washes are required if NH_4Cl solution has been used—Wash cells twice in EMEM containing 10% heat-inactivated human AB serum and resuspend in about 3 ml of this medium. Mix well and transfer 4 drops to a small test tube for cell counting and viability testing. Count cells using Neubauer chamber and Dahl pipette containing cell suspension diluted 1 : 20 in 2.5% acetic acid—Assess viability by mixing equal volumes of cell suspension and 0.4% trypan blue and leave in a waterbath at 37°C for 10 min. Transfer to a slide or counting chamber, add coverslip and allow to settle for 3 min. Count 100 cells, noting the number of blue (dead) cells. Viable cells have not taken up the dye. Calculate the percentage of viable cells. Normally this should be about 95%. If not the method of cell separation should be reviewed.

Mitomycin treatment. Divide each person's cells into two batches. One batch is left untreated. The other batch labelled 'm' will be treated with mitomycin C solution (1 mg/ml PBS). Resuspend cells at 2×10^6/ ml and add 50 μl mitomycin C/ml of cells. Mix well. Incubate mitomycin-treated cells at 37°C, mixing with gentle agitation on Roto-torque, for 30 min. Wash mitomycin-treated cells $\times 3$ in fresh media (EMEM with 10% heat-inactivated AB serum) and resuspend at 2×10^6/ml for addition to culture as stimulator cells. Resuspend untreated cells at 1×10^6/ml for addition to culture as responder cells.

Mixed lymphocyte culture plate. Use plates with round bottomed wells and adopt the following notation:

Patient recipient $= R$
Donors $= D_1, D_2, D_3$ etc.
Mitomycin-treated $= Rm, D_1m, D_2m, D_3m$ etc.

To each test well add 100 μl (2×10^5 cells) of stimulator cells and 100 μl (10^5 cells) of responder cells. Each combination is set up in quadruplicate, except viability wells which are single. Culture the untreated recipient cells with m-treated recipient cells and with each batch of m-treated donor cells, *i.e.* $R + Rm$, $R + D_1m$ etc. This is the basis of the one-way MLC test. Culture each individual's batch of m-treated cells separately to monitor effectiveness of mitomycin treatment, *i.e.* Rm, Dm etc. If sufficient cells are available the following cultures may also be set up. Culture the untreated donor cells with the m-treated recipient cells. Culture both m-treated donor and recipient cells together to monitor effectiveness of mitomycin treatment, *i.e.* $Rm + D_1m$. It is also helpful to culture cells from unrelated donors against each other as a measure of an incompatibility response, *i.e.* $D_1 + D_4m$, $D_1m + D_4$. MLC plates are incubated at 37°C in humid air with 5% CO_2 for six days and pulsed on the fifth day with 2 μC ^3H thymidine 16–20 h before harvesting. Harvest cells onto fibre glass discs using a multiple cell harvester. Dry discs in oven at

60°C for $1\frac{1}{2}$ h. Place discs in scintillation vials in sequence. Add 10 ml of scintillation fluid and count vials in scintillation counter.

Calculation. Results in counts/min may be used to assess the response of recipient to lymphocytes of individual donors.

$$\text{Stimulation index (SI)} = \frac{R + DM}{R + Rm}$$

$$\text{Relative response (RR)} = \frac{(R + Dm) - (R + Rm)}{(R + Xm) - (R + Rm)}$$

$R + Xm$ is the mean of all the recipients' responses to allogeneic cells.

Comment

Albrechtsen et al (1978) used a one-way MLC test in which a relative response (RR) above 30% was taken to indicate definite HLA-D disparity between donor and patient whereas an RR under 15% was taken to indicate HLA-D compatibility. This study of 62 recipients of renal transplants from living relatives mismatched for one or two HLA and/or B antigens indicated a relatively good chance of graft survival (87% survived one year) in patients with a low MLC response compared with a 55% graft survival in the HLA-D incompatible group.

In a similar study Cerilli et al (1978) found that 50% of transplant patients with a high stimulation index (SI > 5) rejected their graft within three months in contrast to 6.5% of patients with a low stimulation index (SI < 5).

The use of MLC in the selection of unrelated donors is controversial and Cullen et al (1977) did not find the test helpful in predicting the graft outcome in 40 cadaveric grafts.

PHYTOHAEMAGGLUTININ STIMULATION

As a measure of cell viability and responsiveness to mitogenic stimulation, cultures from each individual may be set up with phytohaemagglutinin (PHA). The reduced responsiveness of mitomycin-treated cells may also be monitored.

PHA cultures are performed in triplicate in flat-bottomed wells containing 0.1 ml lymphocyte suspension (2×10^6 cells/ml) in Eagles minimum essential medium supplemented with 20 mM glutamine, 50 u penicillin/ml, 50 µg streptomycin/ml, 10 µg gentamycin/ml, 10% foetal calf serum and buffered with 10 mM sodium bicarbonate and 12.5 mM Hepes. PHA is diluted in EMEM at concentrations of 10, 20, 40 and 80 µl/ml and 0.1 ml is added to the well.

PHA plates are incubated for four days and pulsed after 92 h with 0.4 µCi ^{3}H thymidine 4 h before harvesting.

$$\text{PHA stimulation index} = \frac{\text{stimulated-unstimulated cpm}}{\text{unstimulated cpm}}$$

MONITORING THE TRANSPLANT PATIENT

The possibility of allograft rejection is always present in the transplant patient who has received a kidney from a donor who is not an identical twin.

Postoperative progress can be monitored by a variety of functional, biochemical and immunological tests. Elevation of the plasma creatinine although not specific has been found to be a useful indication of the onset of graft rejection.

Hemmingsen et al (1978) have reported on the value of the measurement of the relative clearances of transferrin, haptoglobin, IgG and IgA in the detection of acute rejection episodes. Graft rejection could be predicted up to five days in advance. The predictability of a negative response was 99%, and that of a positive response was 86% rising to 95% if a preceding rise in the urinary excretion of β2 microglobulin was used to exclude false positives. The test was carried out on an auto-analyser and depends on an immunoprecipitin reaction measured by fluornephelometry.

Much effort has been spent on seeking immunological tests which will detect and predict graft rejection episodes. There are different forms of rejection, as outlined in Chapter 7 involving humoral and cellular immunological mechanisms and it is not likely that one particular immunological test will be satisfactory in all cases. *See* review by Ting et al (1978).

Studies have ranged widely from the detection of humoral and cell-mediated cytotoxic activity against donor cells to measurement of lymphocyte populations, responses to mitogens and the detection of antibodies reacting with vascular endothelium.

No test has won widespread acceptance and the reader is referred to the summary by Dossetor & Myburgh (1978) of the First International Symposium on Immunologic Monitoring of the Transplant Patient.

MONITORING IMMUNOSUPPRESSION

With a few exceptions transplant patients require immunosuppression. Unfortunately this predisposes to the development of infection which not only complicates the clinical management of the patient but may result in death.

It would be of considerable advantage to have available a test which would monitor the state of immunosuppression so that a level could be maintained which hopefully was sufficient to avoid allograft rejection but did not unduly predispose to infection.

Some workers have used the T-lymphocyte sheep erythrocyte rosette test to adjust the dose of antithymocyte globulin in individual transplant patients and have found that mainenance at a level of 10% of normal rosetting cells was desirable (Cosimi et al, 1978).

Sheep erythrocyte rosette formation (T lymphocytes)

Equipment
Test tubes 12 × 75 mm—Pipettes: 25 μl; 50 μl—Pasteur pipettes—Microscope slides and coverslips—Microscope—Refrigerator 4°C—Waterbath at 37°C—Centrifuge.

Reagents
Dulbecco A phosphate-buffered saline (pH 7.3, PBS).
Foetal calf serum. (FCS). Heat at 56°C for 30 min to inactivate complement

and absorb with washed sheep erythrocytes for 1 h at 37°C and 1 h at 4°C; centrifuge for 10 min at 1000 g and store at 4°C.

Sheep erythrocytes. Collect in Alsever's solution and store at 4°C for up to two weeks. Before use wash twice in PBS and adjust to 0.5% (v/v) suspension in 50% PBS/absorbed FCS.

Clear fingernail varnish.

Specimen

Lymphocytes are isolated from peripheral blood on a Ficoll-Hypaque gradient and after cell count and assessment of viability are suspended in absorbed FCS at a concentration of 2×10^6 cells/ml.

See Mixed Lymphocyte Culture for lymphocyte separation technique.

Method

(*i*) Add 0.2 ml of the lymphocyte suspension to 0.2 ml of the prepared erythrocyte suspension in a round-bottomed test tube. Cap and place in a waterbath at 37°C for 15 min.

(*ii*) Centrifuge at 200 g for 5 min and place in refrigerator at 4°C overnight for 18 h.

(*iii*) Resuspend the sheep cells by rotating the test tube gently between the palms of the hands. Place one drop of the suspension on a microscope slide and apply a cover slip.

(*iv*) Leave at room temperature for approximately 30 min for excess fluid to evaporate and seal with clear fingernail varnish. Place on microscope and count 200 mononuclear cells. Express the number associated with sheep erythrocyte rosettes as a percentage of the total. A rosette is signified by the presence of three or more sheep erythrocytes adherent to a lymphocyte.

Staining the suspension with 1% toluidine blue for 5 min prior to mounting aids in the identification of lymphocytes in the centre of rosettes and assists in distinguishing rosettes from miscellaneous aggregates of erythrocytes.

Comment

The normal range of sheep erythrocyte rosette-forming cells must be estimated for each laboratory. The mean for our laboratory is 70% and rises to 75% if erythrocytes are pretreated with neuraminidase.

REFERENCES

Albrechtsen D, Flatmark A, Jervell J, Halvorsen S, Solheim B G, Thorsby E 1978 Significance of HLA-D/DR matching in renal transplantation. Lancet 2: 1126–1127

Cerilli J, Williams M A, Newhouse Y G, Fesperman D P 1978 Correlation of tissue typing, mixed lymphocyte culture, and related donor renal allograft survival. Transplantation 26: 218–220

Cosimi A B, Delmonico F L, Burdick J F, Russell P S 1978 Individualized management of immunosuppression according to serial monitoring of immunocompetance. Transplantation Proceedings 10: 647–650

Cullen P R, Lester S, Rouch J, Morris P J 1977 Mixed lymphocyte reaction and graft survival in forty cadaveric renal transplants. Clinical and Experimental Immunology 28: 218–222

Dossetor J B, Myburgh J A 1978 Post-transplant immunologic monitoring: summation. Transplantation Proceedings 10: 661–670

Hemmingsen L, Jensen H, Jest P, Skaarup P 1978 The diagnostic value of protein clearances in rejection of human renal allografts. Acta Medica Scandinavica 203: 107–112

Lobo P I, Westervelt F B, Rudolf L E 1977 Kidney transplantability across a positive cross-match. Cross-match assays and distribution of B lymphocytes in donor tissues. Lancet 1: 925–928
Sheehy M J, Bach F H 1976 Primed LD typing (PLT)—Technical considerations. Tissue Antigens 8: 157–171
Terasaki P I, Bernoco D, Park M S, Ozturk G, Iwaki Y 1978 Microdroplet testing for HLA-A, -B, -C and -D antigens. American Journal of Clinical Pathology 69: 103–120
Ting A, Williams K A, Morris P J 1978 Transplantation: Immunological monitoring. British Medical Bulletin 34: 263–270
Rood J J Van, Balner H, Morris P J 1978 Blood transfusion and transplantation. Transplantation 26: 275–277

INDEX